The LEAN CO

CW01523306

The Simple Sci_____ __ _____ Lean: A Practical Guide to Weight Loss and Muscle Building

A fact-based, no-nonsense approach to transforming your body without gym membership

Table of Contents

Introduction: Why This Book Exists

You don't need another fad diet book. You don't need expensive supplements, fancy gym equipment, or a complete lifestyle overhaul. What you need is the truth about how your body actually works, backed by real science, delivered in a way that makes sense.

This book exists because the weight loss industry has made simple concepts unnecessarily complicated. The science of losing fat and building muscle hasn't changed much in the past 20 years, but the marketing noise has gotten louder. We're going to cut through that noise.

If you're reading this, you're probably somewhere between "slightly frustrated" and "completely fed up" with your current body composition. Maybe you've tried various diets, maybe you've started and stopped gym memberships, or maybe you're just tired of feeling like you need a PhD in nutrition to figure out what to eat for lunch.

Here's what this book will do for you: give you the tools to lose weight, build lean muscle, and maintain both without turning your life upside down.

Chapter 1: The Modern Diet Disaster - How We Got Here

This chapter explains how the typical Western diet evolved into its current state and why it's working against your body composition goals. We'll look at the dramatic shifts in food processing, portion sizes, and eating patterns that have occurred over the past 50 years.

The average person today eats a radically different diet than their grandparents did. While our great-grandparents might have eaten 20-30% of their calories from protein, 30-40% from fats, and the remainder from carbohydrates (mostly from vegetables and whole grains), today's typical Western diet flips this completely upside down.

Modern dietary surveys consistently show that the average American or European now gets about 50- 60% of their calories from carbohydrates, primarily refined ones. Protein intake has dropped to around 15-20% of total calories, while fat intake hovers around 30-35%. But here's the kicker: the quality of all three macronutrients has deteriorated significantly.

Every recommendation is based on peer-reviewed research from the last two decades but explained like you're talking to a knowledgeable friend over coffee.

This isn't about perfection. It's about progress. Let's get started.

The Carbohydrate Explosion

In 1970, the average American consumed about 120 grams of added sugars per year. By 2020, that number had skyrocketed to over 150 pounds annually. That's roughly 400 calories of pure sugar every single day, on top of the natural sugars found in fruits and vegetables.

The rise of processed foods means that carbohydrates now come primarily from refined sources: white bread, pasta, breakfast cereals, and snack foods. These foods are engineered to be hyperpalatable, meaning they trigger reward pathways in your brain that make you want to eat more, even when you're not hungry.

The Breakfast Cereal Scam

Let's talk about breakfast cereals, because they perfectly illustrate how we've been nutritionally bamboozled. Walk down any cereal aisle and you'll see boxes covered in health claims: "Fortified with vitamins!" "Whole grain!" "Heart healthy!" What you're actually looking at is candy disguised as a healthy breakfast.

Most breakfast cereals contain 10-15 grams of sugar per serving. That's 3-4 teaspoons of pure sugar. But here's the dirty secret the serving sizes listed on cereal boxes are laughably small. The box might say "3/4 cup" as a serving, but most people pour at least 1.5 cups into their bowl, doubling the sugar and calorie content before they even add milk.

Cereals exist for one reason: profit margins. Corn, wheat, and rice are incredibly cheap commodities. By processing them into flakes, puffs, and shapes, then adding sugar, artificial colors, and synthetic vitamins, food companies can sell 50 cents worth of grain for $5. They've convinced three generations of parents that this sugar delivery system is not just acceptable, but necessary for a "balanced breakfast."

The marketing is brilliant and insidious. They slap a few vitamins on the side of the box and suddenly it's "fortified." They use whole grain flour (along with three types of sugar) and call it "wholesome." They sponsor studies showing that "cereal eaters have lower Body Mass Indexes" without mentioning that people who eat cereal for breakfast also tend to eat fewer calories throughout the day because they're following diet programs that include portion-controlled cereal as a meal replacement.

Research published in the American Journal of Clinical Nutrition shows that people eating diets high in refined carbohydrates experience blood sugar spikes and crashes that directly trigger hunger hormones, leading to overeating by an average of 300-500 calories per day. Breakfast cereals are particularly problematic because they set you up for this cycle from the moment you wake up.

The Protein Problem

While our ancestors might have gotten protein from whole animals, eggs, and dairy, modern protein sources are often highly processed and combined with additional calories from fats and carbohydrates. A piece of grilled chicken breast is pure protein with minimal calories. A chicken nugget is protein wrapped in refined flour, vegetable oil, and preservatives.

Studies from the International Journal of Obesity demonstrate that people consuming less than 1.2 grams of protein per kilogram of body weight (a common scenario in modern diets) lose significantly more muscle mass during weight loss attempts, making it harder to maintain their new weight long-term.

The Fat Confusion

The low-fat diet craze of the 1980s and 1990s didn't make people thinner. Instead, it led to the replacement of natural fats with refined carbohydrates and artificial additives. When you remove fat from food, you must replace it with something to maintain taste and texture. That something is usually sugar, salt, or chemical flavor enhancers.

Ironically, research from the New England Journal of Medicine shows that people following moderate-fat diets (30-35% of calories) lose weight more effectively and maintain that loss better than those on low-fat diets.

Portion Size Reality Check

The portions we consider "normal" today would have been considered enormous just 40 years ago. A medium McDonald's fries in 1970 contained 200 calories. Today's medium fries contain 340 calories. A typical bagel has grown from 140 calories to over 350 calories.

This "portion creep" affects everything we eat, including supposedly healthy foods. Restaurant salads now average 730 calories, and a typical muffin contains 400-600 calories - more than many people should eat for an entire meal.

The Convenience Trap

The final piece of our modern dietary disaster is the prioritization of convenience over nutrition. We've created a food system where the fastest, easiest options are almost always the worst for your body composition. You can get 2,000 calories of processed food delivered to your door in 30 minutes, but finding 200 calories of quality protein might require a trip to three different stores.

This isn't an accident. The foods that make you gain weight are also the foods with the highest profit margins and the longest shelf lives. Fresh vegetables spoil. Packaged cookies can sit in a warehouse for months. Guess which one gets more marketing dollars and shelf space?

Understanding how we got here is the first step in getting out. The good news? You don't need to completely overhaul your life. You just need to understand what actually works and why.

Chapter 2: The GLP-1 Revolution - A Game-Changing Breakthrough

This chapter celebrates one of the most significant medical breakthroughs in weight management history and explains how this book complements GLP-1 therapy, especially for maintaining results after treatment ends.

Something remarkable has happened in the world of weight loss medicine. For the first time in history, we have medications that work with your body's natural hunger and satiety signals to help you lose significant weight safely and effectively. These medications, called GLP-1 receptor agonists, represent the biggest breakthrough in obesity treatment since we started understanding the science of metabolism.

What Are GLP-1 Medications?

GLP-1 (glucagon-like peptide-1) is a hormone your body naturally produces in your intestines after you eat. It tells your brain "I'm full" and slows down how quickly food leaves your stomach. It also helps regulate blood sugar by stimulating insulin production when needed.

The breakthrough came when researchers figured out how to create synthetic versions of this hormone that last longer in your body. Medications like semaglutide (Ozempic, Wegovy) and tirzepatide (Mounjaro, Zepbound) are essentially giving your body's natural appetite control system a major upgrade.

Clinical trials show average weight losses of 15-20% of body weight - results that were previously only achievable through bariatric surgery. For a 200-pound (91 kg) person, that's 30-40 pounds (14-18 kg) of weight loss. More importantly, people maintain this weight loss as long as they stay on the medication.

Why This Is Revolutionary (And Why You Should Celebrate It)

Let's be clear about something: if GLP-1 medications are available to you and appropriate for your situation, they're not cheating. They're not a shortcut. They're correcting a biological system that, for many people, has been working against them their entire lives. Obesity is NOT a function of whether a person is LAZY or not despite how it is stigmatized. Two individuals who eat the exact same diet and do the same physical activity can have drastically different body shapes. I believe GLP1 drugs will be recorded in history as one of the greatest scientific breakthroughs of this century.

The obesity epidemic isn't a moral failing or a lack of willpower. It's largely the result of evolutionary biology meeting modern food engineering. Your ancestors never had to resist the temptation of hyperpalatable processed foods designed by teams of food scientists to trigger overeating. GLP-1 medications help level that playing field.

Research published in Nature Medicine shows that people with obesity often have dysregulated hunger hormones, including insufficient GLP-1 production. These medications aren't giving you superpowers - they're restoring normal function to your appetite control system.

Where This Book Fits In

Here's the reality about GLP-1 medications: they're incredibly effective for weight loss, but they don't teach you what to do with that weight loss. They don't automatically build muscle, improve your relationship with food, or create sustainable lifestyle habits.

More importantly, many people won't stay on these medications forever. Insurance coverage varies, side effects can be challenging for some, and others simply prefer not to be on long-term medication. The

research shows that when people stop GLP-1 medications without having developed sustainable habits, they regain most of the weight they lost.

That's where this book becomes invaluable. Whether you're currently taking GLP-1 medications, planning to start them, or preparing to transition off them, the principles in this book will help you:

- Maximize muscle preservation during weight loss

- Develop eating patterns that support long-term weight maintenance

- Build physical activity habits that don't require a gym membership

- Understand your body composition beyond just the number on the scale

- Create sustainable routines that work with your real life

The Perfect Partnership

Think of GLP-1 medications as giving you the

breathing room to learn and implement better habits. When you're not constantly fighting hunger and cravings, you have the mental and emotional space to focus on nutrition quality, meal timing, and building lean muscle mass.

The combination of GLP-1 therapy with the evidence-based strategies in this book isn't just additive - it's synergistic. The medication handles the appetite regulation while you build the knowledge and habits that will serve you for life.

Studies from the Diabetes, Obesity and Metabolism journal show that people who combine GLP-1 medications with structured lifestyle interventions (exactly what this book provides) lose more weight and maintain it better than those using medication alone.

Looking Forward

The GLP-1 breakthrough has fundamentally changed the conversation around weight loss. We're moving away from blame and shame toward treating obesity as the complex metabolic condition it actually is.

This book exists in that new paradigm - not as a replacement for medical intervention when appropriate,

but as a complement to it.

Whether you're using GLP-1 medications now, might use them in the future, or are managing your weight through lifestyle changes alone, the science-based strategies in the following chapters will help you achieve and maintain the healthy, strong body you want. Let's dive into that science.

Chapter 3: Macronutrients Decoded - Carbs, Protein, and Fat Explained

This chapter breaks down the three macronutrients in simple terms, explaining what they do in your body and how they affect weight loss and muscle building. We'll debunk common myths and give you the practical knowledge you need to make better food choices.

Your body runs on three types of fuel: carbohydrates, proteins, and fats. Think of them like different types of gasoline for your car. They all provide energy, but they burn differently, cost different amounts, and affect your engine's performance in distinct ways.

Carbohydrates: The Quick Burn Fuel

Carbohydrates are your body's preferred source of quick energy. They break down into glucose (blood sugar) faster than any other macronutrient. This can be good or bad, depending on the type and timing.

There are two main types of carbohydrates: simple and complex. Simple carbs (sugars) hit your bloodstream fast, causing a spike in insulin and a quick burst of energy followed by a crash. Complex carbs (starches and fiber) break down more slowly, providing steadier energy.

Here's what you need to know for weight loss: your body can only store about 400-500 grams (14-18 oz) of carbohydrates as glycogen in your muscles and liver. Anything beyond that gets converted to fat for storage. This process is efficient and automatic.

The current dietary guidelines suggest 45-65% of your calories should come from carbohydrates. For someone eating 2,000 calories per day, that's 225-325 grams (8-11.5 oz) of carbs daily. But research from the Journal of the American Medical Association shows that people lose weight more effectively when they reduce carbohydrate intake to 20-30% of total calories while increasing protein.

Protein: The Body Builder

Protein is different. While carbs and fats are primarily fuel sources, protein is your body's construction material. Every muscle fiber, enzyme, hormone, and antibody in your body is made from protein. When you eat protein, your body breaks it down into amino acids, which are like individual Lego blocks that can be reassembled into whatever your body needs.

Here's the key point for weight loss: protein has the highest thermic effect of all macronutrients. This means your body burns more calories just digesting and processing protein than it does with carbs or fat. About 25-30% of the calories in protein are burned during digestion, compared to 6-8% for carbs and 2-3% for fat.

Protein also triggers the release of hormones that make you feel full and satisfied, reducing your appetite for hours after eating. Studies consistently show that people who increase their protein intake naturally eat 200-400 fewer calories per day without consciously trying to restrict food.

Fat: The Misunderstood Macronutrient

For decades, we were told that dietary fat makes you fat. This is like saying that eating yellow foods makes you yellow. Fat is actually essential for hormone production, brain function, and the absorption of fat-soluble vitamins (A, D, E, and K).

Fat provides 9 calories per gram (compared to 4

calories per gram for protein and carbs), making it the most calorie-dense macronutrient. This is why portion control matters more with fats than with other nutrients. But don't let that scare you away from eating fat - your body needs it.

The key is choosing the right types of fat. Monounsaturated fats (olive oil, avocados, nuts) and omega-3 fatty acids (fish, walnuts, flaxseed) support health and don't interfere with weight loss. Trans fats and excessive omega-6 oils (found in most processed foods) can promote inflammation and make weight loss harder.

The Ideal Macronutrient Split for Weight Loss

Based on the current research, here's what works best for most people trying to lose weight and build lean muscle:

- **Protein: 25-35% of total calories** (this is much higher than standard recommendations, and we'll explain why in the next chapter)

- **Fat: 25-35% of total calories** (focusing on healthy sources)

- **Carbohydrates: 30-50% of total calories**

(emphasizing vegetables, fruits, and minimal processed foods)

For a person eating 2,000 calories per day, this would translate to:

- Protein: 125-175 grams (4.4-6.2 oz)
- Fat 56-78 grams (2-2.8 oz)
- Carbohydrates: 150-250 grams (5.3-8.8 oz)

This isn't about being perfect every day. It's about understanding the general framework so you can make better choices consistently over time.

Chapter 4: Protein is King - The Foundation of Your New Body

This chapter explains why protein deserves the starring role in your nutrition plan and provides specific recommendations for how much you should eat based on your goals and target weight.

If you remember nothing else from this book, remember this: protein is the most important macronutrient for changing your body composition. It's not just important - it's absolutely critical. Here's why, and more importantly, here's exactly how much you need.

Why Protein Rules Everything

Protein does four things that make it indispensable for weight loss and muscle building:

1. **It burns calories just being digested.**
   Remember the thermic effect we mentioned? About 25-30% of protein calories are burned during digestion. If you eat 100 calories of protein, your body automatically burns 25-30 of those calories processing it. Eat 100 calories of sugar, and you only burn 6-8 calories processing

it.

2. **It kills your appetite.** Protein triggers the release of peptide VY, GLP-1 (yes, the same hormone in those breakthrough medications), and other hormones that signal satiety to your brain. A study in the American Journal of Clinical Nutrition found that people who increased their protein intake from 15% to 30% of calories naturally ate 441 fewer calories per day without consciously restricting food.

3. **It preserves muscle during weight loss.** When you're in a calorie deficit, your body will break down both fat and muscle for energy. Higher protein intake significantly reduces muscle loss. Research shows that people eating 0.7 grams per pound (1.6g per kg) of body weight retain 2-3 times more muscle during weight loss compared to those eating lower amounts.

4. **It requires energy to build and maintain muscle.** Muscle tissue is metabolically active, burning calories 24/7. Every pound of muscle burns approximately 6-10 calories per day at rest. That might not sound like much, but over time it adds up to significant differences in how many calories you can eat without gaining

weight. The more muscle you have the easier it is to keep the fat off.

How Much Protein Do You Actually Need?

Here's where most nutrition advice fails you. The RDA (Recommended Dietary Allowance) for protein is 0.36 grams per pound (0.8g per kg) of body weight. This amount prevents protein deficiency diseases. It does not optimize body composition, muscle building, or weight loss.

For weight loss and muscle building, the research is clear: **you need significantly more protein**. Here are the evidence-based recommendations:

For Weight Loss (preserving muscle while losing fat):

- **0.7-1.0 grams per pound of target body weight (1.6-2.2g per kg)**

For Muscle Building (gaining lean mass):

- **0.8-1.2 grams per pound of target body weight** (1.8-2.6g per kg)

For People Over 40 (counteracting age-related muscle loss):

- **1.0-1.2 grams per pound of target body weight**

(2.2-2.6g per kg)

Notice I said "target body weight," not current body weight. If you weigh 200 pounds (91 kg) but want to weigh 160 pounds (73 kg), base your protein intake on 160 pounds (73 kg). This prevents you from eating excessive calories while ensuring adequate protein for your goal physique.

Real-World Examples

Let's make this practical with some examples:

Sarah: Currently 180 lbs (82 kg), wants to weigh 140 lbs (64 kg)

- Target protein intake: 98-140 grams per day (3.5-4.9 oz)

- This equals 4-6 palm-sized portions of protein spread throughout the day

Mike: Currently 220 lbs (100 kg), wants to weigh 180 lbs (82 kg)

- Target protein intake: 126-180 grams per day (4.4-6.3 oz)

- This equals 5-7 palm-sized portions of protein spread throughout the day

Lisa (age 45): Currently 160 lbs (73 kg), wants to maintain weight but build muscle

- Target protein intake: 160-192 grams per day (5.6-6.8 oz)

- This equals 6-7 palm-sized portions of protein spread throughout the day

The Practical Protein Plan

Here's how to hit these numbers without obsessing over every gram:

1. **Eat protein at every meal.** Aim for 25-40 grams (1-1.4 oz) per meal if you eat three meals, or 20-30 grams (0.7-1.1 oz) per meal if you eat four meals.

2. **Use your palm as a guide.** A palm-sized portion of most protein sources provides about 25-30 grams (1-1.1 oz) of protein.

3. **Start your day with protein.** Having 30-40 grams (1.1-1.4 oz) of protein at breakfast sets you up for better appetite control all day.

4. **Don't forget liquid protein.** Protein shakes, Greek yogurt, and milk can help you reach your targets, especially post-workout.

What Counts as Protein?

Focus on complete proteins - foods that contain all essential amino acids:

- Meat, poultry, fish, seafood

- Eggs and egg whites

- Dairy products (milk, Greek yogurt, cheese)

- Protein powders (whey, casein, high-quality plant blends)

Incomplete proteins still count toward your total, but shouldn't be your primary sources:

- Beans, lentils, quinoa

- Nuts and seeds (a great snack alternative to chips or chocolate)

- Whole grains

The Bottom Line

Most people dramatically undereat protein. If you're currently eating the standard American diet, you're probably getting 60-80 grams (2.1-2.8 oz) of protein per day. Doubling that intake will likely be the single most effective change you can make for your body composition.

Yes, it requires some planning at first. Yes, it might feel like a lot of food initially. But within 2-3 weeks, your appetite will adjust, and eating adequate protein will feel natural. The results - better satiety, faster fat loss, preserved muscle mass - make it worth the effort.

Chapter 5: Animal vs. Plant Proteins - The Ultimate Showdown

This chapter objectively compares animal and plant protein sources for muscle building and weight loss, focusing on amino acid profiles, caloric efficiency, and practical considerations for real-world meal planning.

Let's settle this debate once and for all, using science instead of ideology. Both animal and plant proteins can support your goals, but they're not identical in their effects on body composition. Here's what you need to know to make informed choices.

The Amino Acid Advantage: Complete vs. Incomplete

Proteins are made up of 20 different amino acids, nine of which are "essential" - your body can't make them, so you must get them from food. Animal proteins contain all nine essential amino acids in ratios that closely match human needs. Plant proteins typically lack one or more essential amino acids or have them in suboptimal ratios.

This matters for muscle building. Research in the

Journal of the International Society of Sports Nutrition shows that consuming all essential amino acids in adequate amounts triggers maximum muscle protein synthesis - the process by which your body builds new muscle tissue.

Leucine: The Muscle-Building Trigger

One amino acid deserves special attention: leucine. It acts like a key that turns on muscle protein synthesis. You need about 2.5-3 grams of leucine per meal to maximally stimulate muscle building.

Here's how different protein sources stack up:

High-Leucine Animal Proteins:

- 6 oz (170g) chicken breast: 2.8g leucine, 165 calories

- 6 oz (170g) lean beef: 2.6g leucine, 180 calories

- 1 cup Greek yogurt: 2.5g leucine, 150 calories

- 3 large eggs: 2.4g leucine, 210 calories

Plant Proteins (per serving needed to reach 2.5g leucine):

- 1.5 cups cooked quinoa: 2.5g leucine, 330 calories

- 1.5 cups cooked lentils: 2.5g leucine, 340 calories

- 2 cups cooked black beans: 2.5g leucine, 450 calories

- 3 oz (85g) tofu: 1.8g leucine (insufficient alone), 180 calories

Caloric Efficiency: Getting More Protein for Fewer Calories

This is where animal proteins shine brightest. When you're trying to lose weight, every calorie matters. Getting adequate protein while staying in a calorie deficit is much easier with animal sources.

Protein per Calorie Champions:

- Egg whites: 11g protein per 50 calories

- White fish (cod, tilapia): 22g protein per 100 calories

- Chicken breast: 27g protein per 130 calories

- Lean turkey: 26g protein per 120 calories

- Non-fat Greek yogurt: 20g protein per 100 calories

Plant Protein Sources:

- Lentils: 189 protein per 230 calories

- Black beans: 15g protein per 225 calories

- Quinoa: 89 protein per 220 calories

- Tofu: 20g protein per 180 calories (best plant option)

- Tempeh: 31g protein per 320 calories

Absorption and Utilization

Your body doesn't absorb and use all proteins equally. This is measured by something called the Protein Digestibility-Corrected Amino Acid Score (PDCAAS), where 1.0 is perfect:

Animal Protein PDCAAS Scores:

- Whey protein: 1.0

- Egg protein: 1.0

- Milk protein: 1.0

- Beef: 0.92

- Fish: 1.0

Plant Protein PDCAAS Scores:

- Soy protein isolate: 1.0

- Quinoa: 1.0
- Black beans: 0.75
- Peanuts: 0.52
- Wheat: 0.25

The Plant Protein Strategy

If you prefer plant proteins for ethical, environmental, or health reasons, you can absolutely build muscle and lose weight effectively. Here's how to optimize plant protein intake:

1. **Combine complementary proteins.** Rice and beans, hummus and pita, or peanut butter and whole grain bread create complete amino acid profiles.

2. **Focus on the highest-quality plant proteins.** Soy products (tofu, tempeh, edamame), quinoa, and hemp seeds are your best options.

3. **Consider plant protein powder.** High-quality plant protein blends (pea + rice + hemp) can match animal proteins for amino acid completeness and muscle-building effects.

4. **Eat more total protein.** Since plant proteins are less efficiently used, aim for the higher end of the protein recommendations - 1.0-1.2

grams per pound (2.2-2.6g per kg) of target
body weight.

S. **Time your plant proteins strategically.** Have
your highest-quality plant proteins (tofu,
tempeh, protein powder) around your
workouts when muscle protein synthesis is
elevated.

Mixed Approach: The Best of Both Worlds

Many people find success with a flexible approach
that includes both animal and plant proteins. This
might look like:

- **Breakfast:** Greek yogurt with berries (animal
protein)

- **Lunch:** Large salad with chickpeas and hemp
seeds (plant protein)

- **Snack:** Protein shake with plant-based powder

- **Dinner:** Grilled fish with quinoa and vegetables
(animal + plant)

This approach maximizes amino acid variety while
maintaining caloric efficiency for weight loss goals.

The Verdict

For pure muscle-building efficiency and weight
loss support, animal proteins have clear

advantages in amino acid completeness, leucine content, and caloric efficiency. However, well-planned plant-based diets can absolutely support excellent body composition results.

The best protein is the one you'll consistently eat. If you love plants, eat plants - just be strategic about it. If you prefer animal proteins, include them - just choose lean sources most of the time. If you like both, use both strategically based on your daily calorie and protein targets.

Chapter 6: Timing is Everything - When to Eat for Maximum Results

This chapter explores the science of meal timing, intermittent fasting, and post-workout nutrition to help you optimize when you eat for better fat loss, muscle building, and appetite control.

The fitness industry loves to overcomplicate meal timing. You've probably heard that you need to eat every 2-3 hours to "stoke your metabolic fire" or that eating after 8 PM automatically turns food into fat. Most of this is nonsense. But some aspects of when you eat do matter for optimizing your results.

The Metabolism Myth: Meal Frequency Doesn't Matter Much

Let's start by destroying the biggest meal timing myth: that eating more frequently boosts your metabolism. Multiple studies, including a comprehensive review in the British Journal of Nutrition, show that eating 6 small meals versus 3 larger meals has no significant effect on metabolic rate, fat loss, or muscle preservation.

Your body's thermic effect of food (the calories burned digesting meals) depends on total food intake, not meal frequency. Whether you eat 2,000 calories in 2 meals or 6 meals, you'll burn roughly the same number of calories processing that food.

This is liberating. You don't need to carry around Tupperware containers or set phone alarms to eat every few hours. Eat when it's convenient and fits your lifestyle.

What Actually Matters: The 4 Timing Principles That Work

1. Protein Distribution Throughout the Day

While total daily protein is most important, spreading it across meals does matter for muscle building. Your muscle protein synthesis response peaks at about 25-30 grams (1-1.1 oz) of high-quality protein per meal, then plateaus.

This means eating 100 grams (3.5 oz) of protein in one meal isn't twice as effective as eating 50 grams (1.8 oz). You'll get better muscle-building results from 4 meals with 25 grams (0.9 oz) each than from 2 meals with 50 grams (1.8 oz) each.

Practical application: Aim for 20-40 grams (0.7-1.4 oz) of protein per meal, distributed relatively evenly throughout your eating window.

2. Post-Workout Nutrition (The 2-Hour Window)

The "anabolic window" - the idea that you must eat protein within 30 minutes of working out - has been grossly exaggerated. Research shows you actually have about 2 hours post-workout when your muscles are primed to use protein for building and repair.

If you've eaten protein within 3-4 hours before your workout, you don't need to panic about immediate post-workout nutrition. Your blood amino acid levels are still elevated. However, if you work out first thing in the morning or haven't eaten protein in several hours, having 25-40 grams (0.9-1.4 oz) of protein within an hour of finishing your workout is beneficial.

3. Pre-Sleep Protein

Your body builds and repairs muscle while you sleep, but this process requires available amino acids. Having 20-30 grams (0.7-1.1 oz) of slow-digesting protein (like Greek yogurt or casein protein) 1-2 hours before bed can support overnight muscle building and recovery.

Studies show that people who eat protein before bed gain more muscle and lose more fat compared to those who stop eating earlier in the evening, assuming total daily calories and protein are matched.

4. Carbohydrate Timing for Energy and Recovery

Carbohydrates are best consumed when your body can use them immediately for energy or to replenish glycogen stores. The optimal times are:

- **Before workouts:** 30-50 grams (1.1-1.8 oz) of carbs 1-2 hours before exercise can improve performance

- **After workouts:** 30-60 grams (1.1-2.1 oz) of carbs post-workout helps replenish muscle glycogen

- **Earlier in the day:** You're more insulin sensitive in the morning, making carbs less likely to be stored as fat

Intermittent Fasting: Useful Tool or Overhyped Trend?

Intermittent fasting (IF) has exploded in popularity, with claims ranging from "miraculous fat loss" to "fountain of youth effects." The reality is more nuanced.

What intermittent fasting actually does:

- Makes it easier to maintain a calorie deficit by restricting your eating window

- May improve insulin sensitivity and metabolic flexibility

- Simplifies meal planning and can reduce total daily calories without conscious restriction

What intermittent fasting doesn't do:

- Provide magical fat-burning benefits beyond calorie restriction

- Boost metabolism significantly

- Work better than other calorie-matched approaches for fat loss

The most studied and practical IF approach is the 16:8 method - fasting for 16 hours and eating within an 8-hour window. This often means skipping breakfast and eating from noon to 8 PM, or eating breakfast and skipping dinner.

Who benefits from intermittent fasting:

- People who naturally prefer fewer, larger meals

- Those who struggle with constant snacking

- Busy individuals who find meal planning easier with fewer meals

- People who feel more energetic when fasting

Who should avoid intermittent fasting:

- Anyone with a history of eating disorders

- People taking medications that require food

- Those who feel weak, dizzy, or overly hungry when fasting

- Pregnant or breastfeeding women

The Late-Night Eating Myth

"Don't eat after 8 **PM**" is one of the most persistent diet myths. Your body doesn't have a magical cutoff time when calories suddenly count double. Weight gain happens when you consistently eat more calories than you burn, regardless of timing.

However, there are practical reasons why late-night eating often leads to weight gain:

- Evening snacks are usually high-calorie, processed foods

- People tend to eat mindlessly while watching TV or relaxing

- Late meals can interfere with sleep quality

- Eating large meals close to bedtime can cause digestive discomfort

The solution isn't to avoid eating after an arbitrary time. It's to plan your evening eating just like your daytime eating, focusing on protein and vegetables if you're hungry at night.

Your Personal Timing Strategy

The best meal timing is the one that helps you consistently hit your protein and calorie targets while fitting your lifestyle. Here are three effective approaches:

Traditional 3-Meal Approach:

- Breakfast: 25-35g (0.9-1.2 oz) protein

- Lunch: 25-35g (0.9-1.2 oz) protein

- Dinner: 25-35g (0.9-1.2 oz) protein

- Optional evening snack: 15-209 (0.5-0.7 oz) protein

16:8 Intermittent Fasting:

- 12 PM: 30-40g (1.1-1.4 oz) protein

- 4 PM: 20-30g (0.7-1.1 oz) protein snack

- 7 PM: 35-45g (1.2-1.6 oz) protein

4-Meal Approach:

- Breakfast: 20-25g (0.7-0.9 oz) protein

- Lunch: 25-30g (0.9-1.1 oz) protein

- Afternoon snack: 15-20g (0.5-0.7 oz) protein

- Dinner: 25-30g (0.9-1.1 oz) protein

The Bottom Line on Timing

Focus on hitting your daily protein and calorie targets first. Once you've mastered that, you can optimize timing for small additional benefits. The perfect timing plan that you can't stick to is worthless. The good enough timing plan that you follow consistently will transform your body.

Chapter 7: The Food Villains - What's Actually Sabotaging Your Progress

This chapter identifies the specific foods and eating patterns that make weight loss unnecessarily difficult, explaining why they're problematic and offering practical strategies for avoiding or managing them.

Not all foods are created equal when it comes to your body composition goals. Some foods work with your biology to support satiety, stable energy, and lean muscle building. Others work against you, triggering overeating, energy crashes, and fat storage. Let's identify the real villains in your diet.

The Hyperpalatable Food Trap

The biggest dietary villains aren't necessarily the ones you expect. It's not butter (a natural fat) or even sugar (at least you know what it is). The real villains are hyperpalatable foods - products engineered by food scientists to trigger overconsumption by hitting your "bliss point" of salt, sugar, and fat

Research from the University of Michigan identified the most addictive foods based on their ability to trigger loss of control eating. The top offenders combine multiple rewarding ingredients in ways that don't exist in nature:

The Worst Offenders:

- Pizza (combines refined carbs, cheese, processed meat, and oil)

- Chocolate (sugar + fat in perfect addiction ratios)

- Chips (salt + oil + refined carbs with engineered crunch)

- Cookies (sugar + refined flour + fat)

- Ice cream (sugar + fat + cold temperature reward)

- French fries (starch + oil + salt with satisfying texture)

These foods bypass your natural satiety signals. You can easily eat 1,000+ calories of chips or cookies without feeling satisfied, but try eating 1,000 calories of chicken breast and vegetables - it's nearly impossible.

Ultra-Processed Foods: The 70% Problem

Ultra-processed foods now make up about 70% of the American food supply. These are products that have been broken down into component parts and reassembled with additives, preservatives, and flavor enhancers. They're designed for shelf stability and profit margins, not your health.

A landmark study published in Cell Metabolism had people eat either ultra-processed foods or whole foods for two weeks, with meals matched for calories, protein, fat, carbs, and fiber. The ultra-processed group ate an average of 508 more calories per day and gained 2 pounds (0.9 kg), while the whole foods group lost 2 pounds (0.9 kg).

Examples of ultra-processed villains:

- Breakfast cereals (even "healthy" ones)
- Granola bars and protein bars (most of them)
- Flavored yogurts with mix-ins
- Instant oatmeal packets
- Frozen meals and convenience foods
- Most bread (check the ingredient list - real bread has 4-5 ingredients)
- Salad dressings and condiments
- Plant-based meat substitutes (often highly processed despite health halo)

The Liquid Calorie Catastrophe

Your brain doesn't register liquid calories the same way it registers solid food calories. You can drink a 400-calorie frappuccino and still eat a full meal an hour later, but eating 400 calories of solid food would significantly reduce your appetite for the next meal.

Liquid calorie villains:

- **Specialty coffee drinks:** A venti Starbucks Frappuccino contains 400-500 calories

- **Smoothies:** Even "healthy" smoothies often pack 300-600 calories with multiple servings of fruit

- **Juices:** Orange juice has more sugar per ounce than Coca-Cola

- **Sports drinks:** Unnecessary unless you're exercising intensely for over an hour

- **Alcohol:** We'll cover this extensively in the next chapter

- **Protein shakes with additions:** That "healthy" smoothie with protein powder, banana, peanut butter, and milk can easily hit 600+ calories

The "Health Halo" Deceptions

Some of the worst dietary villains hide behind health claims. These foods make you feel virtuous while sabotaging your progress:

Granola and Trail Mix: Often 500+ calories per cup with added sugars and oils. A small handful can pack 200 calories.

Dried Fruit: All the sugar of fresh fruit concentrated into tiny portions. A quarter cup of dried cranberries has as much sugar as a candy bar.

Nut Butters: Natural and healthy, but also 190 calories per 2-tablespoon serving. Easy to underestimate portions.

Avocado: Nutritious but calorie-dense at 250-300 calories per medium avocado. Instagram's favorite toast topping can easily hit 400+ calories.

Quinoa and Ancient Grains: Healthy but not magical. Still 220 calories per cooked cup, same as white nee.

"Keto" Packaged Foods: Often just regular junk food with different ingredients, still engineered for overconsumption.

Restaurant Portion Distortion

Even "healthy" restaurant choices can sabotage your progress through sheer portion size:

- **Restaurant salads:** Often 800-1,200 calories with dressing, cheese, nuts, and croutons

- **Grilled chicken entrees:** The 8-12 oz (225-340g) portions common in restaurants are 2-3 times what most people need

- **"Small" sides:** Restaurant side portions are often larger than home main courses

- **Hidden fats:** Restaurant food uses far more oil and butter than home cooking

The Snacking Trap

Constant snacking, even on "healthy" foods, can prevent weight loss by keeping insulin levels elevated and providing continuous calories. The worst snacking patterns include:

- **Mindless munching:** Eating while distracted by TV, work, or phones

- **Emergency snacking:** Keeping "healthy" snacks everywhere "just in case"

- **Fruit overload:** Treating fruit as "free" food and eating unlimited quantities

- **Nut addiction:** Going through a bag of almonds while convincing yourself they're healthy

Identifying Your Personal Food Villains

Everyone has specific trigger foods that lead to overeating. Common patterns include:

1. **The "Just One" Foods:** You tell yourself you'll have just one cookie/chip/piece of candy but end up eating the whole package

2. **The Stress Eaters:** Specific foods you turn to when tired, stressed, or emotional

3. **The Social Saboteurs:** Foods you only

   overeat in certain situations (office parties,

   happy hours, family gatherings)

4. **The Convenience Crutches:** Processed foods you rely on when busy or unprepared

Practical Villain Management Strategies

You don't need to eliminate all these foods forever, but you do need strategies for managing them:

For hyperpalatable foods:

- Don't keep them in your house

- If you buy them, buy single servings only

- Plan when and where you'll eat them (conscious indulgence vs. mindless consumpton)

For liquid calories:

- Drink water, tea, and black coffee as primary beverages

- If you drink calories, account for them in your daily total

- Have protein-rich foods with liquid calories to improve satiety

For health halo foods:

- Read nutrition labels, notjust marketing claims

- Measure portions of calorie-dense "healthy" foods

- Ask "Would I eat this much if it weren't considered healthy?"

For restaurant foods:

- Check nutrition information online before going

- Ask for dressing and sauces on the side

- Consider sharing entrees or saving half for later

The goal isn't perfection. It's awareness. When you understand which foods make your goals harder to achieve, you can make informed decisions about when and how to include them in your life.

Chapter 8: The Alcohol Truth - Liquid Calories and Your Waistline

This chapter provides an honest, science-based look at how alcohol affects weight loss, muscle building, and metabolism, plus practical strategies for those who choose to drink while pursuing body composition goals.

Let's have an honest conversation about alcohol and your body composition goals. This isn't about being preachy or telling you to become a teetotaler. It's about understanding exactly how alcohol affects your progress so you can make informed decisions.

How Alcohol Affects Your Body Composition

Alcohol is metabolically unique. It's not quite a carbohydrate, not quite a fat, but it provides 7 calories per gram (almost as much as fat's 9 calories per gram). More importantly, your body treats alcohol as a toxin that must be processed immediately, which creates a cascade of effects that work against your goals.

The Metabolic Shutdown Effect

When you drink alcohol, your liver stops virtually

everything else to focus on breaking down the alcohol. This means:

- **Fat burning stops:** Your body can't burn fat while processing alcohol

- **Protein synthesis decreases:** Muscle building is impaired for up to 24 hours after drinking

- **Blood sugar regulation suffers:** Your liver can't properly manage glucose while dealing with alcohol

Studies published in the American Journal of Clinical Nutrition show that just two drinks can reduce fat burning by up to 73% for several hours. If you're trying to lose fat, this is a significant metabolic roadblock.

The Appetite Destruction

Alcohol doesn't just add calories - it makes you eat more calories from other sources. Research consistently shows that people consume 200-500 additional food calories on days they drink alcohol compared to non-drinking days.

This happens through multiple mechanisms:

- **Lowered inhibitions:** You're more likely to say "screw it" and order the nachos

- **Disrupted hunger hormones:** Alcohol interferes with leptin and ghrelin signaling

- **Blood sugar crashes:** Alcohol can cause delayed hypoglycemia, triggering intense food cravings

- **Dehydration confusion:** Your body sometimes mistakes thirst for hunger

The Sleep and Recovery Sabotage

Quality sleep is crucial for muscle building, fat loss, and hormone regulation. Alcohol systematically destroys sleep quality:

- **Reduced REM sleep:** The restorative sleep phase when growth hormone is released

- **Increased sleep fragmentation:** More wake-ups during the night

- **Dehydration effects:** Leading to poor sleep quality and morning fatigue

- **Disrupted melatonin:** Your natural sleep-wake cycle gets thrown off

Even if you feel like you're sleeping the same amount after drinking, the quality is significantly reduced. Poor sleep leads to increased cortisol, reduced testosterone and growth hormone, and impaired recovery from exercise.

The Calorie Reality Check

Most people drastically underestimate alcohol calories. Here's the reality:

Beer (12 oz/355ml):

- Light beer: 100-110 calories

- Regular beer: 140-170 calories

- IPA/Craft beer: 180-250 calories

- Imperial stouts: 250-350+ calories

Wine (5 oz/1SOml):

- White wine: 120-130 calories

- Red wine: 125-135 calories

- Sweet wines: 140-170 calories

- Fortified wines: 165-180 calories

Spirits (1.5 oz/45ml):

- Vodka, gin, rum, whiskey: 95-100 calories

- Liqueurs: 160-200+ calories

Mixed Drinks:

- Margarita: 300-500 calories

- Pina colada: 400-600 calories

- Long Island iced tea: 500-700 calories

- Moscow mule: 200-250 calories

The Hidden Calories in "Low-Calorie" Drinks

Even drinks marketed as healthier options can sabotage your progress:

- **Wine spritzers:** Still 80-120 calories plus often high in sugar

- **Spiked seltzers:** 90-110 calories, but easy to drink many

- **Light cocktails:** Often use artificial sweeteners that may trigger cravings

- **Skinny" versions:** Usually just smaller portions or different mixers, still significant calories

The Muscle Building Interference

If you're trying to build muscle, alcohol creates several problems:

Protein Synthesis Impairment: Studies show that alcohol consumption reduces muscle protein synthesis by 15-20% for up to 24 hours, even when adequate protein is consumed.

Hormone Disruption: Alcohol temporarily reduces testosterone levels and increases cortisol, both of which interfere with muscle building and fat loss.

Nutrient Displacement: Alcohol calories are "empty" -

they provide energy but no vitamins, minerals, or amino acids needed for muscle building.

Dehydration Effects: Proper hydration is crucial for muscle function and recovery. Alcohol is a diuretic that promotes fluid loss.

Practical Strategies for Social Drinkers

If you choose to drink while pursuing body composition goals, here are evidence-based strategies to minimize the damage:

Strategy 1: Account for the Calories

- Track alcohol calories just like food calories
- Consider reducing food calories on drinking days (but not protein)
- Plan your drinks in advance rather than drinking impulsively

Strategy 2: Choose Your Timing

- Avoid drinking on workout days when possible
- If you must drink post-workout, wait at least 2-3 hours
- Don't drink on consecutive days to allow recovery

Strategy 3: Optimize Your Choices

- Stick to straight spirits with zero-calorie mixers (vodka soda, whiskey neat)

- Choose dry wines over sweet wines

- Avoid beer if calories are a major concern (worst calorie-to-alcohol ratio)

- Alternate alcoholic drinks with water

Strategy 4: Minimize the Food Damage

- Eat a protein-rich meal before drinking to slow alcohol absorption

- Have healthy snacks available to avoid drunk food choices

- Plan your post-drinking meal in advance

Strategy 5: Damage Control

- Drink extra water before, during, and after alcohol consumption

- Take a multivitamin on drinking days to replace depleted nutrients

- Get as much quality sleep as possible

- Don't skip your workout the next day (even if it's lighter than usual)

The 80/20 Approach to Alcohol

For most people, the most sustainable approach is moderation rather than elimination. This might look like:

- **80% of the time:** Minimal or no alcohol (1-2 drinks per week max)
- **20% of the time:** Social drinking occasions where you plan and account for it

This allows you to maintain your social life and enjoy occasional drinks without completely derailing your progress.

When to Consider Eliminating Alcohol Completely

Some people benefit from cutting out alcohol entirely while pursuing body composition goals:

- **Fast results needed:** If you have a specific deadline or event
- **Struggling with cravings:** If alcohol triggers overeating
- **Poor sleep quality:** If you're already struggling with recovery
- **Medication interactions:** Always follow medical advice
- **Personal preference:** If you simply don't miss it

The Bottom Line on Booze

Alcohol isn't necessarily incompatible with your body composition goals, but it definitely makes them harder to achieve. Every drink is a choice between immediate pleasure and your longer-term goals. Neither choice is inherently right or wrong, but both have consequences.

If you choose to drink, do it consciously and strategically. Account for the calories, minimize the frequency, and have damage control strategies in place. Your progress may be slower, but it doesn't have to stop completely.

If you choose not to drink, you'll likely see faster results and better recovery. The choice is yours, but now you have the information to make it intelligently.

Chapter 9: If You Must - Better Choices for Real Life

This chapter acknowledges that perfection isn't realistic and provides specific substitutions for common indulgences, focusing on harm reduction rather than elimination for sustainable long-term success.

Life happens. Birthday parties, work happy hours, late-night cravings, and moments when you just want something that tastes good. This chapter isn't about being perfect - it's about being strategic when you're not going to be perfect.

The Harm Reduction Philosophy

Traditional diet advice often takes an all-or-nothing approach: either you're "good" and eating grilled chicken with steamed broccoli, or you're "bad" and might as well eat everything in sight. This thinking leads to diet cycles and yo-yo weight patterns.

A more sustainable approach is harm reduction - making the best available choice in any given situation. Sometimes the best choice is a salad. Sometimes the best choice is the smaller portion of pizza instead of the larger one. Both can be "good" choices in context.

Alcohol Substitutions: Still Social, Fewer Calories

When you want to drink but don't want to blow your calorie budget, these swaps can save you 100-300 calories per drink:

Instead of Margaritas (300-500 calories):

- **Choose:** Tequila with fresh lime juice and soda water (110 calories)
- **Savings:** 200-400 calories per drink

Instead of Pina Coladas (400-600 calories):

- **Choose:** White rum with coconut-flavored sparkling water and a splash of pineapple juice (130 calories)
- **Savings:** 270-470 calories per drink

Instead of Beer (140-250+ calories):

- **Choose:** Vodka soda with lime (100 calories)
- **Savings:** 40-150+ calories per drink

Instead of Sweet Wines (140-170 calories):

- **Choose:** Dry wines like Sauvignon Blanc or Pinot Grigio (120 calories)
- **Savings:** 20-50 calories per glass

Instead of Craft Cocktails (200-400+ calories):

- **Choose:** Spirits neat or on the rocks (95-100 calories)
- **Savings:** 100-300+ calories per drink

Smart Mixers That Won't Sabotage You:

- Soda water with fresh citrus
- Diet tonic (if you can tolerate artificial sweeteners)
- Muddled herbs like mint or basil
- A splash of 100% cranberry juice (not cranberry cocktail)
- Kombucha as a mixer for spirits

Snack Swaps: Satisfying Without the Calorie Bomb

Late-night munchies and afternoon cravings don't have to derail your progress. These swaps provide similar satisfaction with fewer calories and better nutrition:

Instead of Potato Chips (150 calories per oz/28g):

- **Choose:** Air-popped popcorn (30 calories per cup) or baked chickpeas (130 calories per oz/28g)

- **Why it works:** You get the crunch and salt satisfaction with more fiber and protein

Instead of Ice Cream (250-400 calories per cup):

- **Choose:** Greek yogurt with frozen berries and a drizzle of honey (150-200 calories per cup)

- **Why it works:** Cold, creamy, sweet, but with 20g protein instead of empty calories

Instead of Cookies (50-150 calories each):

- **Choose:** Apple slices with 2 tbsp almond butter (190 calories total)

- **Why it works:** Sweet, satisfying, but provides fiber, healthy fats, and protein

Instead of Candy (150-250 calories per handful):

- **Choose:** Dates stuffed with nuts (60-80 calories each)

- **Why it works:** Natural sweetness with fiber and healthy fats that actually satisfy

Instead of Crackers with Cheese (200-300 calories per serving):

- **Choose:** Cucumber slices with hummus (100-1SO calories per serving)

- **Why it works:** Same creamy, salty satisfaction with more volume and nutrients

Restaurant Strategies: Eating Out Without Giving Up

You don't need to become a hermit to lose weight. These restaurant strategies help you stay social while staying on track:

Italian Restaurants:

- **Instead of:** Fettuccine Alfredo (1,200+ calories)

- **Choose:** Grilled fish with vegetables and a side of marinara for dipping (400-500 calories)

Mexican Restaurants:

- **Instead of:** Burrito with all the fixings (800-1,200 calories)

- **Choose:** Burrito bowl, no rice, extra lettuce and salsa (400-600 calories)

Asian Restaurants:

- **Instead of:** General Tso's chicken with fried rice (1,000+ calories)

- **Choose:** Steamed chicken and broccoli with brown rice (500-600 calories)

Steakhouses:

- **Instead of:** 16 oz ribeye with loaded potato (1,500+ calories)

- **Choose:** 8 oz filet with grilled asparagus (600-700 calories)

Fast Food Emergencies:

- **McDonald's:** Grilled chicken salad instead of Big Mac meal (saves 600+ calories)

- **Subway:** 6" turkey on whole wheat instead of footlong Italian BMT (saves 500+ calories)

- **Chipotle:** Bowl instead of burrito, skip cheese and sour cream (saves 300+ calories)

Coffee Shop Survival Guide

Your daily coffee habit doesn't have to sabotage your goals:

Instead of Venti Frappuccino (400-500 calories):

- **Choose:** Iced coffee with splash of milk and sugar-free syrup (SO calories)

- **Savings:** 350-450 calories

Instead of Large Latte (220 calories):

- **Choose:** Americana with steamed milk (80 calories)

- **Savings:** 140 calories

Instead of Muffin (400-600 calories):

- **Choose:** Hard-boiled egg and piece of fruit (150 calories)

- **Savings:** 250-450 calories

Party and Event Strategies

Social events don't have to be dietary disasters:

Before the Event:

- Eat a protein-rich snack to avoid arriving hungry

- Decide in advance how many drinks/treats you'll have

- Bring a healthy dish you enjoy to ensure good options

At the Event:

- Fill your plate with vegetables and protein first

- Take small portions of special occasion foods

- Stay hydrated with water between alcoholic drinks

- Focus on socializing rather than grazing

Travel and Convenience Store Options

Stuck at an airport or gas station? These options won't destroy your progress:

Convenience Store Wins:

- Greek yogurt + nuts

- Hard-boiled eggs + apple

- String cheese + jerky

- Protein bars with <5g sugar and >15g protein

Airport Food Court:

- Salad with grilled protein (ask for dressing on the side)

- Sushi rolls (avoid tempura)
- Grilled chicken sandwich, eat half the bun

- Smoothie with protein powder added

The 80/20 Rule in Action

Aim to make optimal choices 80% of the time, and don't stress about the other 20%. This might look like:

- **Monday-Friday:** Structured eating with planned meals and snacks

- **Weekend:** More flexibility for soc al events and

treats

- **Special occasions:** Enjoy yourself without guilt, then get back on track

When Good Enough Is Perfect

Remember, the goal isn't to never eat anything enjoyable again. The goal is to build sustainable habits that allow you to maintain your results long-term. Sometimes "good enough" choices are actually perfect because they prevent the all-or-nothing thinking that leads to giving up entirely.

The best choice is always the one you can live with consistently. Use these substitutions as tools, not rules, and remember that progress beats perfection every single time.

Chapter 10: Beyond BMI - Understanding Body Composition

This chapter explains why body weight alone is misleading and teaches you better ways to track your progress, focusing on body fat percentage, muscle mass, and other meaningful metrics for assessing your health and fitness.

Step away from the scale. No, seriously. The number on your bathroom scale is probably the least informative metric for tracking your body composition progress, yet it's the one most people obsess over. Let's explore better ways to measure what actually matters.

Why BMI Is Basically Useless

Body Mass Index (BMI) was created in the 1830s by a Belgian mathematician - not a doctor, not a nutritionist, but a mathematician looking for population-level statistical correlations. It divides your weight in kilograms by your height in meters squared, giving you a single number that supposedly indicates whether you're healthy.

The problems with BMI are enormous:

It can't distinguish between muscle and fat.
According to BMI, most NFL players are obese. The
Rock (Dwayne Johnson) at 6'5" and 260 lbs (1.96m,
118kg) has a BMI of 31, classifying him as obese.
Meanwhile, someone who is "skinny fat" - normal
weight but high body fat and low muscle mass - gets
classified as healthy.

It ignores body fat distribution. Visceral fat
(around your organs) is dangerous. Subcutaneous
fat (under your skin) is relatively harmless. BMI
can't tell the difference.

It doesn't account for bone density or frame size.
Two people with identical height and weight can
have completely different body compositions based
on bone structure and muscle density.

It fails for different populations. BMI was
developed using data from European populations
and doesn't accurately reflect health risks for
other ethnicities.

What Actually Matters: Body Composition

Instead of focusing on total weight, focus on the ratio
of fat to muscle in your body. Here's why:

Muscle is metabolically active. Every pound of

muscle burns 6-10 calories per day at rest. Every pound of fat burns about 2 calories per day. More muscle means you can eat more food without gaining weight.

Muscle improves function. Stronger muscles mean better posture, fewer injuries, easier daily activities, and maintained independence as you age.

Body fat percentage tells the real story. A 140-pound (64kg) woman with 30% body fat has 42 pounds (19kg) of fat and 98 pounds (44kg) of lean mass. A 160-pound (73kg) woman with 20% body fat has 32 pounds (14.5kg) of fat and 128 pounds (58kg) of lean mass. Who's healthier? The "heavier" woman by every meaningful metric.

Healthy Body Fat Ranges

Here are evidence-based body fat percentage ranges for health and aesthetics:

Men:

- **Essential fat:** 2-5% (athletes only, not sustainable long-term)

- **Athletic:** 6-13% (very lean, visible abs)

- **Fitness:** 14-17% (lean, some ab definition)

- **Average:** 18-24% (healthy but not lean)

- **Obese:** 25%+ (health risks increase significantly)

Women:

- **Essential fat:** 10-13% (needed for normal hormone function)

- **Athletic:** 14-20% (very lean, some ab definition possible)

- **Fitness:** 21-24% (lean, healthy appearance)

- **Average:** 25-31% (healthy but not lean)

- **Obese:** 32%+ (health risks increase significantly)

How to Measure Body Fat Percentage DEXA Scan (Most Accurate):

- Uses X-ray technology to measure bone, muscle, and fat

- Accuracy: ±1-2%

- Cost: $50-150

- Best for: Baseline measurement and tracking major changes

Bod Pod (Very Accurate):

- Uses air displacement to measure body composition

- Accuracy: ±2-3%

- Cost: $40-75
- Best for: Regular tracking if available in your area

Bioelectrical Impedance (Moderately Accurate):

- Sends electrical signals through your body
- Accuracy: ±3-5% (varies greatly with hydration)
- Cost: $25-200 for home scales
- Best for: Tracking trends, not absolute numbers

Skinfold Calipers (Moderately Accurate with Training):

- Measures fat thickness at specific body sites
- Accuracy: ±3-5% with proper technique
- Cost: $10-30
- Best for: Self-tracking if you learn proper technique

Progress Photos and Measurements (Most Practical): While not giving exact body fat percentages, photos and measurements often provide the most motivating and practical feedback:

- **Take photos:** Same lighting, poses, and clothing every 2-4 weeks
- **Measure circumferences:** Waist, hips, arms, thighs monthly

- **Track how clothes fit:** Often more motivating than any number

Why the Scale Lies (And When to Ignore It)

The bathroom scale measures your total relationship with gravity. It doesn't distinguish between:

- **Water weight fluctuations:** Can vary 2-5 lbs (0.9-2.3kg) daily based on sodium, carbs, hormones, and hydration

- **Muscle vs. fat changes:** Muscle is denser than fat, so you can get smaller while weighing the same

- **Digestive contents:** Food and waste in your system can add 1-3 lbs (0.5-1.4kg)

- **Timing factors:** You weigh more at night than in the morning

When the scale goes up but you're doing everything right:

- You started strength training (muscle gain + water retention)

- You're a woman near your menstrual cycle (hormonal water retention)

- You ate more sodium or carbs than usual (temporary water retention)

- You're constipated (happens with dietary changes)

- You're building muscle faster than losing fat (body recomposition)

Better Ways to Track Progress

The Waist-to-Hip Ratio: Measure your waist at its narrowest point and your hips at their widest. Divide waist by hips.

- **Men:** Below 0.90 is healthy, below 0.85 is excellent
- **Women:** Below 0.80 is healthy, below 0.75 is excellent

This ratio predicts health risks better than BMI because it accounts for dangerous visceral fat around your organs.

The Clothes Test: Pick a piece of clothing that's currently snug but not impossible to wear. Try it on every 2-3 weeks. How it fits is often more meaningful than scale weight.

Energy and Performance Markers:

- Can you climb stairs without getting winded?
- Do you have more energy throughout the day?
- Are you sleeping better?
- Can you lift heavier weights or walk farther?
- Has your mood improved?

The Monthly Check-In System

Instead of daily scale obsession, try this monthly assessment:

Week 1: Take progress photos and measurements
Week 2: Try on your "test" clothes **Week 3:** Get a body fat measurement (if accessible) **Week 4:** Weigh yourself once, in the morning, after using the bathroom

This gives you multiple data points while preventing daily scale fluctuations from derailing your motivation.

Body Recomposition: The Holy Grail

The most impressive transformations often happen when people maintain their weight while simultaneously losing fat and gaining muscle. This is called body recomposition, and it's particularly common when:

- You're new to strength training
- You significantly increase your protein intake
- You're in your first year of consistent exercise
- You're a man under 35 or a woman under 30

During recomposition, the scale might not budge for months, but you'll look dramatically different. Your clothes will fit better, you'll see muscle definition, and your body fat percentage will drop significantly.

Setting Realistic Expectations Healthy fat loss rates:

- **Beginners:** 1-2 lbs (0.5-0.9kg) per week for the first month

- **Ongoing:** 0.5-1 lb (0.2-0.5kg) per week for most people

- **Last 10-15 lbs:** 0.25-0 5 lb (0.1-0.2kg) per week (it gets slower)

Muscle building rates:

- **Beginners:** 1-2 lbs (0.5-0.9kg) per month for the first 6 months

- **Intermediate:** 0.5-1 lb (0.2-0.5kg) per month

- **Advanced:** 0.25-0.5 lb (0.1-0.2kg) per month

The Bottom Line on Body Composition

Your scale weight is just one piece of data, and often not the most important one. Focus on building muscle, losing fat, and improving your health markers. The aesthetic results you want will follow naturally.

Remember: a 140-pound (64kg) woman with 25% body fat looks completely different from a 140-pound woman with 18% body fat. The second woman will appear leaner, stronger, and more defined despite weighing exactly the same.

Stop letting a number on a scale determine your self-worth. Start focusing on the composition of that number, and you'll be amazed at what your body can achieve.

Chapter 11: The Calorie Equation - Input vs. Output Simplified

This chapter explains the fundamental energy balance equation for weight loss and weight gain, debunking myths while providing practical strategies for managing your caloric intake and expenditure.

Weight loss and weight gain ultimately come down to one fundamental equation: calories in versus calories out. This isn't the whole story, but it's the foundation that everything else builds upon. Let's break down this equation and make it work for you.

The First Law of Thermodynamics (AKA Reality)

Your body obeys the laws of physics. Energy cannot be created or destroyed, only transformed. If you consume more energy (calories) than you expend, the excess gets stored as fat. If you expend more energy than you consume, your body breaks down stored fat (and sometimes muscle) to make up the difference.

This is not negotiable. It's not influenced by your metabolism type, your genetics, or your blood type. It's as reliable as gravity.

But it's not that simple in practice...

While the calorie equation is fundamental, several factors influence both sides of the equation in ways that make real-world application more complex:

Calories In: It's Not Just About the Number

The Thermic Effect of Food varies by macronutrient:

- **Protein:** 20-30% of calories burned during digestion
- **Carbohydrates:** 5-10% of calories burned during digestion
- **Fats:** 0-3% of calories burned during digestion

This means 100 calories of chicken breast only provides about 75 net calories to your body, while 100 calories of butter provides about 98 net calories.

Food quality affects satiety and adherence: 100 calories of almonds will keep you satisfied much longer than 100 calories of candy, making it easier to maintain your calorie deficit.

Gut bacteria influence calorie absorption: Some people extract more calories from the same foods due to differences in intestinal bacteria populations.

Calories Out: More Complex Than You Think

Your total daily energy expenditure (TDEE) consists of four components:

1. Basal Metabolic Rate (BMR) - 60-75% of total calories The energy required to keep you alive at rest. This includes:

- Brain function (about 20% of your BMR)
- Heart, lungs, kidneys, liver function
- Cellular maintenance and repair
- Protein synthesis

2. Thermic Effect of Food (TEF) - 8-15% of total calories The energy cost of digesting, absorbing, and processing food.

3. Exercise Activity Thermogenesis (EATI - 15-30% of total calories Planned physical activity: gym workouts, sports, running, etc.

4. Non-Exercise Activity Thermogenesis (NEAT) - 15-50% of total calories All movement that isn't planned exercise:

- Fidgeting, gesturing, maintaining posture
- Occupational activities (typing, walking around

office)

- Daily life activities (cooking, cleaning, shopping)

Why Metabolic Adaptation Happens

When you eat fewer calories for an extended period, your body adapts to preserve energy:

BMR decreases by 10-25%: Your body becomes more efficient at basic functions **NEAT decreases significantly:** You unconsciously move less throughout the day **TEF decreases:** Less food means less thermic effect **Exercise becomes more efficient:** You burn fewer calories doing the same workouts

This is why weight loss often stalls after several months, even when you're eating the same calories that previously caused weight loss.

Calculating Your Caloric Needs Step 1: Estimate Your BMR

For Men: BMR = 88.362 + (13.397 $\times$ weight in kg) + (4.799 $\times$ height in cm) - (5.677 $\times$ age)

For Women:

BMR = 447.593 + (9.247 $\times$ weight in kg) + (3.098 $\times$ height in cm) - (4.330 $\times$ age)

Quick conversions:

- Pounds to kg: divide by 2.2

- Inches to cm: multiply by 2.54

Step 2: Multiply by Activity Factor

- **Sedentary (office job, no exercise):** BMR x 1.2

- **Lightly active (light exercise 1-3 days/week):** BMR x 1.375

- **Moderately active (moderate exercise 3-5 days/week):** BMR x 1.55

- **Very active (hard exercise 6-7 days/week):** BMR x 1.725

- **Extremely active (hard exercise+ physical job):** BMR x 1.9

Example Calculation: Saran: 34 years old, 165 lbs (75kg), 5'6" (168cm), lightly active

BMR = 447.593 + (9.247 x 75) + (3.098 x 168) - (4.330 x 34)

BMR = 447.593 + 693.525 + 520.464 - 147.22 = 1,514 calories

TDEE = 1,514 x 1.375 = 2,082 calories per day

Creating Your Calorie Deficit

For sustainable fat loss, create a deficit of 500-750

calories per day, which should result in 1-1.5 lbs (0.5-0.7kg) of weight loss per week.

Sarah's weight loss plan:

- TDEE: 2,082 calories
- Deficit target: 500-600 calories
- Daily calories for weight loss: 1,400-1,500

The 80/20 Rule for Calorie Management

You don't need to be perfect with calories every single day. Aim for:

80% of days: Hit your calorie target within 100 calories

20% of days: Allow flexibility for social events, special occasions, or just life happening

Your weekly average matters more than daily perfection.

Practical Calorie Management Strategies

1. Track for Awareness, Not Obsession

- Use a food tracking app for 2-4 weeks to learn portion sizes
- Focus on hitting protein targets first, then total calories
- Don't stress about being exactly precise every day

2. Use the Plate Method

- ½ **plate:** Non-starchy vegetables
- ¼ **plate:** Lean protein (palm-sized portion)
- ¼ **plate:** Complex carbohydrates or healthy fats
- This naturally creates appropriate portions for most people

3. Calorie Banking If you know you'll eat more on weekends, eat 100-200 fewer calories Monday through Friday and "bank" those calories for weekend social events.

4. The Two-Day Rule If you overeat significantly one day, get back on track the next day. Don't try to "make up for it" by eating extremely little - this usually backfires.

Common Calorie Counting Mistakes

Underestimating portions: Most people underestimate their food intake by 20-40%. Measure portions occasionally to recalibrate your estimates.

Forgetting liquid calories: Drinks, cooking oils, and condiments add up quickly and are often forgotten.

Weekend amnesia: Tracking perfectly Monday-Friday

then eating freely on weekends can wipe out your entire weekly deficit.

Overestimating exercise calories: Fitness trackers and gym machines often overestimate calorie burn by 15-25%.

Not accounting for bites, licks, and tastes: That spoonful of peanut butter, those few chips while cooking, the sample at the grocery store - it all adds up.

When Calories Aren't Everything

While calorie balance drives weight loss, other factors influence body composition and health:

Meal timing can optimize results: Eating protein throughout the day supports muscle maintenance **Food quality affects satiety:** Whole foods keep you satisfied longer than processed foods **Hormone optimization matters:** Adequate sleep and stress management support healthy metabolism **Muscle preservation is crucial:** Strength training and adequate protein prevent metabolic slowdown

Breaking Through Plateaus

When weight loss stalls despite maintaining your

calorie deficit:

Option 1: Reduce calories by 100-150 per day Option 2: Increase daily activity (more walking, take stairs, etc.) Option 3: Add 1-2 additional strength training sessions per week Option 4: Take a 1-2 week diet break at maintenance calories

The Bottom Line on Calories

Calories matter. They're not the only thing that matters, but they're the foundation that everything else builds upon. You can't out-supplement a poor diet, you can't out-exercise a terrible diet, and you can't

ignore the laws of thermodynamics.

But you also don't need to count every calorie for the rest of your life. Use calorie awareness as a tool to reach your goals, then transition to intuitive eating patterns that maintain your results.

The goal is to understand the calorie equation well enough that managing your weight becomes automatic, not obsessive.

Chapter 12: No Gym, No Problem - The Science of Home Fitness

This chapter proves that effective weight loss and muscle building don't require expensive gym memberships or fancy equipment, backed by research on bodyweight training and home workout effectiveness.

The fitness industry wants you to believe that you need a $50+ monthly gym membership, personal trainers, and expensive equipment to get in shape. This is marketing, not science. Some of the fittest people in the world - military personnel, gymnasts, martial artists - build their foundation using primarily bodyweight exercises.

The Research on Home Workouts

A landmark study published in the American Journal of Health Promotion followed 100 overweight adults for 6 months. Half used a traditional gym membership, half did home-based bodyweight workouts. The results were virtually identical for weight loss, muscle gain, and cardiovascular improvement.

Another study in the Journal of Sports Medicine and

Physical Fitness compared bodyweight training to weight training for muscle development. After 8 weeks, both groups showed similar improvements in muscle strength and endurance, with the bodyweight group actually showing superior improvements in functional movement patterns.

Why Home Workouts Work

Consistency beats intensity. The best workout is the one you'll actually do. Home workouts eliminate common barriers:

- No commute time (saves 20-30 minutes per session)
- No waiting for equipment
- No gym intimidation or social anxiety
- Works with any schedule, any weather
- Zero ongoing costs after initial setup

Progressive overload is still possible. You can make bodyweight exercises harder by:

- Increasing repetitions
- Slowing down the movement tempo
- Adding pauses or holds
- Progressing to more challenging variations

- Reducing rest time between exercises

Compound movements rule. The best home exercises work multiple muscle groups simultaneously, providing maximum benefit in minimum time. Push-ups work chest, shoulders, triceps, and core. Squats work legs, glutes, and core. Pull-ups work back, biceps, and core.

Equipment-Free Exercise Science

Bodyweight Squats for Lower Body: Research shows that bodyweight squats activate the quadriceps, hamstrings, and glutes as effectively as weighted squats for the first 12-15 repetitions. For most beginners and intermediates, this provides sufficient stimulus for muscle development and strength gains.

Push-ups for Upper Body: A study in the Journal of Strength and Conditioning Research found that push-ups performed at different angles (feet elevated, hands elevated, standard) can target muscles as effectively as bench pressing different weights. The beauty is built-in progression: wall push-ups _, knee push-ups _, full push-ups _, decline push-ups _, one-arm push-ups.

Planks for Core Stability: Electromyography (EMG) studies show that planks activate core muscles more comprehensively than traditional crunches or sit-ups. A 60-second plank activates the deep stabilizing muscles that protect your spine during daily activities.

The Metabolic Benefits

High-intensity bodyweight circuits create an "afterburn effect" (excess post-exercise oxygen consumption) that continues burning calories for hours after your workout ends. A study in the European Journal of Applied Physiology found that a 20-minute high-intensity bodyweight circuit burned as many total calories over 24 hours as a 40-minute moderate-intensity treadmill session.

The Psychology of Home Success

Lower barrier to entry: When your workout space is 10 feet away instead of a 20-minute drive, you're 3-4 times more likely to exercise consistently.

Privacy and comfort: Many people, especially beginners, feel self-conscious in gyms. Home workouts eliminate this barrier entirely.

Family integration: Home workouts can include family members, making fitness a shared activity rather than time away from loved ones.

Habit formation: Research on habit formation shows that reducing friction (making things easier) dramatically increases adherence. Home workouts eliminate most friction from the exercise equation.

Setting Up Your Home Fitness Space

You need surprisingly little space

and equipment to create an

effective home gym: **Minimum**

Space Required: 6 feet x 6 feet

(1.8m x 1.8m) of clear floor space

Essential Equipment (under

$100 total):

- Yoga/exercise mat ($15-30)
- Resistance bands set ($15-25)
- Suspension trainer or TRX-style system ($30-50)
- Optional: Set of dumbbells or kettlebell ($20-40)

Advanced Equipment (if budget allows):

- Pull-up bar ($20-40)

- Adjustable dumbbells ($100-200)
- Stability ball ($15-25)

Bodyweight Exercise Progressions:

Push-up Progression:

1. Wall push-ups (hands against wall)
2. Incline push-ups (hands on couch/chair)
3. Knee push-ups
4. Full push-ups
5. Decline push-ups (feet elevated)
6. Single-arm push-ups

Squat Progression:

1. Chair-assisted squats
2. Bodyweight squats
3. Jump squats
4. Single-leg squats (pistol squats)
5. Squat holds and pulses

Core Progression:

1. Dead bugs and bird dogs

2. Modified planks (knees down)

3. **Full** planks

4. Side planks

5. Plank variations (up-down, mountain climbers)

The Home Cardio Solution

Effective cardiovascular exercise doesn't require treadmills or stationary bikes:

Stair Climbing: Walking up and down stairs for 10-15 minutes burns 100-150 calories and improves cardiovascular fitness as effectively as moderate jogging.

Bodyweight Circuits: Alternating between squats, push-ups, mountain climbers, and jumping jacks for 20-30 minutes provides excellent cardiovascular conditioning.

Dancing: 30 minutes of dancing burns 200-300 calories while improving coordination and mood. Put on music and move - it counts as cardio.

Household Chores: Vigorous cleaning, gardening, and yard work can burn 150-300 calories per hour while accomplishing necessary tasks.

The Walking Prescription

The simplest and most underrated form of exercise is walking. Research consistently shows that people who walk 8,000-10,000 steps per day (about 4-5 miles or 6-8 km) have:

- 35% lower risk of heart disease
- 40% lower risk of type 2 diabetes
- 20% lower risk of premature death
- Better weight management and mood regulation

Making walking work for weight loss:

- Walk for 30-45 minutes daily at a brisk pace
- Add hills or stairs to increase intensity
- Walk after meals to improve blood sugar control
- Use walking as thinking/phone call time to maximize efficiency

Creating Your Home Routine

The Minimal Effective Dose: Research shows that as little as 3 sessions per week, 20-30 minutes each, can produce significant improvements in strength, cardiovascular fitness, and body composition.

Sample Weekly Schedule:

- **Monday:** Upper body bodyweight circuit (20

minutes)

- **Tuesday:** 30-45 minute walk

- **Wednesday:** Lower body and core circuit (20 minutes)

- **Thursday:** Active recovery (gentle yoga, stretching, easy walk)

- **Friday:** Full-body circuit (25 minutes)

- **Saturday:** Longer activity (hiking, dancing, sports with family)

- **Sunday:** Rest or gentle movement

The Accountability Factor

Home workouts require more self-motivation than gym workouts. Strategies for success:

Schedule workouts like appointments: Put them in your calendar and treat them as non-negotiable commitments.

Start small: Begin with 10-15 minute sessions to build the habit before increasing duration.

Track your progress: Keep a simple log of workouts completed and improvements noticed.

Find virtual accountability: Online fitness communities, workout apps, or virtual training sessions with friends.

The Bottom Line on Home Fitness

You don't need a gym membership to transform your body. You need consistency, progressive overload, and the willingness to work hard for 2J-30 minutes several times per week. The equipment and space are nice-to-haves, not necessities.

The best part? Once you've built strength and confidence with home workouts, you can take these skills anywhere. Hotel rooms, parks, friend's houses - your gym travels with you.

Stop using the lack of a gym membership as an excuse. Your body doesn't know whether you're doing push-ups in a fancy fitness center or your living room. It only knows whether you're challenging it to adapt and grow stronger.

Chapter 13: Quick and Effective - Resistance Training in Minutes

This chapter focuses on time-efficient resistance exercises that build strength and muscle using minimal equipment, perfect for busy schedules and home workouts.

Time is the most common excuse for not exercising. "I don't have an hour to spend at the gym" is what most people think resistance training requires. The truth? You can build significant strength and muscle with just 15-20 minutes of focused resistance training, 3 times per week.

The Science of Minimal Effective Dose

Research from the Journal of Strength and Conditioning Research shows that strength gains plateau after about 45-60 minutes of training. In fact, sessions longer than 60 minutes can actually impair results due to increased cortisol and fatigue.

More importantly, a study published in Medicine & Science in Sports & Exercise found that people doing 15-minute resistance sessions 3 times per week gained 90% as much strength as those doing

45-minute sessions. The key was intensity and focus, not duration.

Why Short Workouts Work

Higher intensity is possible: When you know you only need to work hard for 15 minutes, you can push yourself harder than during longer sessions.

Better recovery: Shorter sessions don't tax your nervous system as heavily, allowing for better recovery and more frequent training.

Easier consistency: It's much easier to find 15 minutes three times per week than 60 minutes three times per week.

Less intimidating: Short workouts feel achievable, reducing the mental resistance that keeps people from starting.

The Big 6: Foundation Movements

Every effective resistance program builds around these six fundamental movement patterns. Master these, and you'll develop balanced strength throughout your entire body:

1. Push (Horizontal) - Push-ups and Variations

- **Muscles worked:** Chest, shoulders, triceps, core

- **Beginner:** Wall push-ups or incline push-ups

- **Intermediate:** Standard push-ups

- **Advanced:** Decline push-ups or single-arm push-ups

2. Push (Vertical) - Pike Push-ups and Handstand Progressions

- **Muscles worked:** Shoulders, triceps, upper chest, core

- **Beginner:** Pike push-ups with feet on ground

- **Intermediate:** Pike push-ups with feet elevated

- **Advanced:** Handstand push-ups against wall

3. Pull (Horizontal) - Rows

- **Muscles worked:** Back, biceps, rear shoulders

- **Equipment needed:** Resistance bands or suspension trainer

- **Beginner:** Assisted rows with feet closer to anchor

- **Intermediate:** Standard rows

- **Advanced:** Single-arm rows or archer rows

4. Pull (Vertical) - Pull-ups and Chin-ups

- **Muscles worked:** Back, biceps, forearms, core

- **Beginner:** Assisted pull-ups with resistance band

- **Intermediate:** Full pull-ups or chin-ups

- **Advanced:** Weighted pull-ups or muscle-ups

5. Squat Pattern - Squats and Variations

- **Muscles worked:** Quadriceps, glutes, hamstrings, core

- **Beginner:** Chair-assisted squats

- **Intermediate:** Bodyweight squats

- **Advanced:** Jump squats or single-leg squats

6. Hinge Pattern - Deadlift Variations

- **Muscles worked:** Hamstrings, glutes, lower back, core

- **Beginner:** Glute bridges

- **Intermediate:** Single-leg deadlifts

- **Advanced:** Broad jumps or single-leg hip thrusts

The 15-Minute Strength Circuit

This circuit hits all major muscle groups in minimal time. Perform 3 rounds, 45 seconds work, 15 seconds rest between exercises, 60 seconds rest between rounds:

Round Structure:

1. Push-ups (or your current progression)

2. Squats

3. Rows (with resistance band/suspension trainer)

4. Plank hold

5. Glute bridges

6. Pike push-ups (or overhead press with resistance band)

Total time: 15 minutes including warm-up and cool-down.

The 1-Minute Miracle Moves
When you have literally one minute, these exercises provide maximum benefit:

1-Minute Plank Challenge:

- Hold a plank for as long as possible

- Rest briefly when needed, continue until 60 seconds total

- Builds core strength, improves posture, engages entire body

1-Minute Push-up Test:

- Perform as many push-ups as possible in 60

seconds

- Use whatever progression level you can maintain good form

- Builds upper body strength and muscular endurance

1-Minute Squat Hold:

- Hold a squat position for as long as possible

- Rest briefly when needed, continue until 60 seconds total

- Builds leg strength, improves hip mobility

1-Minute Wall Sit:

- Back against wall, slide down until thighs parallel to floor

- Hold position for up to 60 seconds

- Builds quadriceps strength and mental toughness

Progressive Overload Without Weights

The key to continued progress is making exercises progressively more challenging:

Increase Repetitions:

- Week 1: 8 push-ups

- Week 2: 10 push-ups

- Week 3: 12 push-ups

Slow Down the Movement:

- 2-second lowering phase

- 1-second pause at bottom

- 2-second raising phase

Add Range of Motion:

- Deficit push-ups (hands on books for deeper stretch)

- Deep squats (full range of motion)

Unilateral Training:

- Single-arm push-ups

- Single-leg squats

- Alternating movements

Add Instability:

- Push-ups with feet on stability ball

- Single-leg stands during upper body exercises

The Isometric Advantage

Holding positions (isometric contractions) builds incredible strength in minimal time:

Plank Progressions (30-60 seconds each):

- Standard plank

- Side planks (both sides)

- Plank with leg lifts

- Plank to push-up position

Wall Sit Progressions:

- Basic wall sit (30-60 seconds)

- Single-leg wall sit

- Wall sit with calf raises

Glute Bridge Holds:

- Double-leg bridge hold (30-60 seconds)

- Single-leg bridge hold

- Bridge with marching

The Resistance Band Solution

Resistance bands provide variable resistance and take up almost no space:

Upper Body Band Circuit (10 minutes):

1. Band pull-aparts

2. Overhead press

3. Rows

4. Bicep curls

5. Tricep extensions

Lower Body Band Circuit (10 minutes):

1. Banded squats

2. Lateral walks

3. Glute bridges with band

4. Standing hip abductions

5. Monster walks

Recovery and Progression

Rest Between Sessions: Allow at least 48 hours between intense resistance sessions for the same muscle groups.

Listen to Your Body: Some muscle soreness is normal, sharp pain is not. Adjust intensity accordingly.

Progress Gradually: Increase difficulty by 10-20% per week maximum. It's better to progress slowly and avoid injury.

Track Your Progress:

- Number of repetitions completed

- How long you can hold isometric positions

- When you graduate to harder exercise variations

The Busy Person's Weekly Plan

Monday - Upper Body Focus (15 minutes):

- Push-ups: 3 sets

- Rows: 3 sets

- Pike push-ups: 2 sets

- Plank: 2 sets

Wednesday - Lower Body Focus (15 minutes):

- Squats: 3 sets

- Glute bridges: 3 sets

- Single-leg deadlifts: 2 sets

- Wall sit: 2 sets

Friday - Full Body Circuit (20 minutes):

- The 15-minute circuit described above

- Plus 5 minutes of stretching

The Bottom Line on Quick Resistance Training

You don't need hours in the gym to build strength and muscle. You need consistency, progressive overload, and the willingness to work intensely for short periods. Fifteen focused minutes beats sixty distracted minutes every time.

The beauty of bodyweight resistance training is that it scales with you. As you get stronger, the exercises get more challenging. As your schedule gets busier, the workouts can get shorter while remaining effective.

Stop waiting for the perfect time to start a comprehensive fitness program. Start with what you have - your body, a small space, and 15 minutes. The strength you build will surprise you.

Chapter 14: Get Your Heart Pumping - Simple Cardio That Works

This chapter provides practical cardiovascular exercise options that burn calories, improve heart health, and complement your strength training - all without expensive equipment or gym memberships.

Cardiovascular exercise doesn't have to mean running on a treadmill for an hour. The best cardio is the kind you'll actually do consistently, and there are dozens of ways to get your heart rate up that don't require a gym membership or expensive equipment.

The Science of Cardio for Weight Loss

Research consistently shows that cardiovascular exercise burns calories during the activity and provides modest increases in metabolism for several hours afterward. However, the real magic happens when you combine cardio with resistance training.

A study in the International Journal of Sport Nutrition found that people who combined moderate cardio with resistance training lost 40% more fat than those who did cardio alone, while preserving significantly more muscle mass.

The key insight: Cardio burns calories now, muscle burns calories forever. The best approach uses cardio to increase your daily calorie deficit while using resistance training to build the muscle that keeps you lean long-term.

Understanding Heart Rate Zones

Your heart rate during exercise determines what type of adaptations your body makes:

Fat-Burning Zone (60-70% max heart rate):

- Easy conversation pace
- Can maintain for 30+ minutes
- Primary fuel source: stored fat
- Examples: Brisk walking, easy cycling

Aerobic Zone (70-80% max heart rate):

- Slightly breathless but sustainable
- Can maintain for 20-60 minutes
- Primary fuel source: mix of fat and carbohydrates
- Examples: Jogging, swimming, cycling at moderate pace

Anaerobic Zone (80-90% max heart rate):

- Hard breathing, can only speak a few words

- Can maintain for 2-20 minutes

- Primary fuel source: stored carbohydrates

- Examples: High-intensity intervals, sprinting

Maximum Effort (90-100% max heart rate):

- All-out effort, no talking possible

- Can maintain for 10 seconds to 2 minutes

- Examples: Sprint intervals, burpees, mountain climbers

Calculating Your Target Heart Rate

Simple formula: 220 - your age = estimated maximum heart rate

Example for a 35-year-old:

- Maximum heart rate: 220 - 35 = 185 beats per minute

- Fat-burning zone: 111-130 bpm (60-70%)

- Aerobic zone: 130-148 bpm (70-80%)

- Anaerobic zone: 148-167 bpm (80-90%)

The Walking Revolution

Walking is the most underrated and accessible form of cardiovascular exercise. Research from Harvard Medical School shows that people who walk regularly have:

- 30-35% lower risk of heart disease

- 40% lower risk of type 2 diabetes

- 20% lower risk of stroke

- Better weight management and mood regulation

The Daily Mile Challenge: Walking just one mile (1.6 km) per day burns approximately 80-100 calories and takes most people 15-20 minutes. Over a year, this single habit could result in 8-10 pounds (3.6-4.5 kg) of weight loss without any other changes.

Making walking work for weight loss:

- **Morning walks:** Boost metabolism and energy for the day

- **Post-meal walks:** Improve blood sugar control and aid digestion

- **Evening walks:** Reduce stress and improve sleep quality
- **Weekend longer walks:** 45-60 minutes for greater calorie burn

Stair Climbing: The Hidden Gem

Stair climbing burns 8-11 calories per minute - more than most other cardio activities. A 10-minute stair climbing session burns 80-110 calories while building leg strength simultaneously.

The Daily Stair Challenge:

- Find a staircase with 10-20 steps
- Walk up and down 10 times
- Total time: 5-10 minutes
- Calories burned: 50-80
- Can be done anywhere: home, office, public buildings

High-Intensity Interval Training (HIIT)

HIIT involves alternating between short bursts of intense activity and periods of rest or low-intensity activity. Research shows HIIT can burn more calories in less time compared to steady-state cardio.

Beginner HIIT Protocol (12 minutes total):

- 3-minute warm-up (easy walking)
- 6 rounds of: 30 seconds hard effort, 30 seconds easy recovery
- 3-minute cool-down

Advanced HIIT Protocol (16 minutes total):

- 3-minute warm-up
- 8 rounds of: 45 seconds hard effort, 15 seconds rest
- 3-minute cool-down

HIIT can be applied to any activity:

- Walking/jogging intervals
- Bodyweight exercise circuits
- Stair climbing intervals
- Swimming intervals
- Cycling intervals

Home Cardio Options

Dancing (200-400 calories per 30 minutes): Put on your favorite music and move. Dancing improves coordination, burns calories, and boosts mood. No special skills required - just move your body to the beat.

Household Chores (150-300 calories per hour):

- Vacuuming vigorously
- Scrubbing floors or bathrooms
- Gardening and yard work

- Washing windows

- Rearranging furniture

Bodyweight Cardio Circuits: Alternate between these exercises for 20-30 minutes:

- Jumping jacks

- Mountain climbers

- Burpees

- High knees

- Butt kickers

- Squat jumps

The Cardio-Strength Combination

The most time-efficient approach combines cardiovascular and strength training:

Circuit Training: Move quickly between resistance exercises with minimal rest. This builds strength while keeping your heart rate elevated.

Example Cardio-Strength Circuit (20 minutes):

1. Push-ups (45 seconds)

2. Jumping jacks (30 seconds)

3. Squats (45 seconds)

4. Mountain climbers (30 seconds)

5. Plank (45 seconds)

6. Burpees (30 seconds)

7. Rest (60 seconds)

8. Repeat 3-4 rounds

Outdoor Cardio Adventures

Hiking: Burns 300-500 calories per hour while providing mental health benefits from nature exposure.

Recreational Sports: Basketball, tennis, soccer, or volleyball burn 400-600 calories per hour while providing social interaction.

Swimming: Low-impact, full-body exercise burning 300-500 calories per hour. Excellent for people with joint issues.

Cycling: Burns 300-600 calories per hour depending on intensity. Can be transportation and exercise combined.

The Consistency Formula

Research shows that people

who exercise consistently

follow these patterns: **Start**

Small: Begin with 10-15

minutes of activity you enjoy,

3 times per week. **Schedule**

It: Treat cardio like an

important appointment. Put it

in your calendar.

Have a Backup Plan: Indoor options for bad weather, short routines for busy days.

Track Progress: Monitor frequency and duration, not just calories burned.

Find Your Why: Connect cardio to goals beyond weight loss (stress relief, energy, sleep quality).

Cardio Mistakes to Avoid

Doing too much too soon: Start with

20-30 minutes, 3 times per week. Build

gradually. **Only doing cardio:** Combine

with resistance training for optimal body

composition results. **Same routine**

every time: Your body adapts quickly.

Vary intensity, duration, and activities.

Ignoring intensity: Moderate effort most of the time, with occasional high-intensity sessions.

Compensating with food: Don't eat back all the

calories you burn. Exercise is for fitness, diet is for

weight loss.

The Bottom Line on Cardio

The best cardiovascular exercise is the one you'll do consistently. Whether it's dancing in your living room, walking around your neighborhood, or playing sports with friends, regular movement that elevates your heart rate will improve your health and support your weight loss goals.

Don't get caught up in finding the "perfect" cardio routine. Start with something you enjoy, do it regularly, and adjust as you get fitter and stronger. Your heart, your waistline, and your mood will thank you.

Chapter 15: What About Me - Real People, Real Plans

This chapter provides specific, actionable plans for different life situations, ages, and goals. Each profile represents real-world scenarios with practical daily recommendations for nutrition, exercise, and realistic timelines for results.

Sometimes the best way to understand how all this science applies to your life is to see how it works for people like you. These profiles represent common situations, complete with specific daily eating plans, exercise routines, and realistic expectations for progress.

SARAH - The Busy Working Mom *Age: 34 | Current: 765 lbs (75kg) | Goal: 740 lbs (64kg) | Timeline: 6-8 months*

Sarah works full-time, has two young kids, and feels like she's gained weight gradually since having children. She wants to lose 25 pounds (11kg) but has maybe 30 minutes per day for herself.

Daily Nutrition Plan:

- **Protein Target:** 98-112 grams (3.5-4 oz) per day

- **Calories:** 1,400-1,500 per day

- **Breakfast:** Greek yogurt (20g protein) with berries and 1 tbsp almond butter (300 calories)

- **Lunch:** Large salad with 4 oz (115g) grilled chicken (30g protein), vegetables, 2 tbsp olive oil dressing (400 calories)

- **Dinner:** 4 oz (115g) salmon with roasted vegetables and small sweet potato (35g protein, 450 calories)

- **Snacks:** String cheese or protein shake if needed (15-20g protein, 150-200 calories)

Daily Exercise (25-30 minutes):

- **3 days/week:** Home resistance circuit (squats, push-ups, planks, lunges) - 15 minutes

- **3 days/week:** Brisk walk while kids play at park or on treadmill while they watch TV - 25 minutes

- **1 day/week:** Rest or gentle yoga

Expected Progress:

- **Weeks 1-2:** 2-3 lbs (1-1.4kg) loss (mostly water weight)
- **Weeks 3-24:** 1-1.5 lbs (0.5-0.7kg) loss per week

- **Final result:** 25 lbs (11kg) lost in 6-7 months

Key Success Strategies:

- Meal prep on Sundays
- Keep protein bars in car/purse for emergencies
- Exercise during kids' screen time or playground visits

MIKE - The Desk Job Dad *Age: 42* | *Current: 275 lbs (98kg)* | *Goal: 785 lbs (84kg)* | *Timeline: 8-10 months*

Mike sits at a computer all day, travels frequently for work, and has developed a "dad bod" over the past decade. He wants to lose 30 pounds (14kg) and build some muscle definition.

Daily Nutrition Plan:

- **Protein Target:** 130-148 grams (4.6-5.2 oz) per day
- **Calories:** 1,800-1,900 per day
- **Breakfast:** 3-egg omelet with vegetables and 1 slice whole grain toast (25g protein, 350 calories)
- **Lunch:** Chipotle-style bowl with double chicken, vegetables, salsa, no rice (45g protein, 500 calories)
- **Dinner:** 6 oz (170g) lean steak with large portion roasted vegetables (40g protein, 550 calories)

- **Snacks:** Protein shake post-workout, apple with 2 tbsp almond butter (25g protein, 350 calories total)

Daily Exercise (35-45 minutes):

- **4 days/week:** Home strength training with basic equipment (resistance bands, dumbbells) - 30 minutes

- **2 days/week:** Cardio (walking, jogging, or stationary bike) - 35 minutes

- **1 day/week:** Active recovery (yard work, hiking with family)

Expected Progress:

- **Weeks 1-2:** 3-4 lbs (1.4-1.8kg) loss

- **Weeks 3-32:** 1-1.5 lbs (0.5-0.7kg) loss per week

- **Final result:** 30 lbs (14kg) lost in 8-9 months, noticeable muscle gain

Key Success Strategies:

- Pack protein-rich snacks for travel

- Use hotel gyms or bodyweight exercises in hotel room
- Meal delivery service for consistent nutrition

JENNIFER - The College Student *Age: 20* | *Current:*

155 lbs (70kg) | *Goal: 135 lbs (61kg)* | *Timeline: 4-5 months*

Jennifer gained the "freshman 15" and wants to lose 20 pounds (9kg) before summer. She has access to a campus gym but limited cooking facilities and a tight budget.

Daily Nutrition Plan:

- **Protein Target:** 95-108 grams (3.4-3.8 oz) per day
- **Calories:** 1,300-1,400 per day
- **Breakfast:** Protein smoothie with protein powder, banana, spinach, almond milk (30g protein, 300 calories)
- **Lunch:** Dining hall salad with grilled chicken, hard-boiled egg, minimal dressing (35g protein, 400 calories)
- **Dinner:** Grilled fish or chicken from dining hall with vegetables (30g protein, 350 calories)
- **Snacks:** Greek yogurt, string cheese, or protein bar (15-20g protein, 150-200 calories)

Daily Exercise (45-60 minutes):

- **3 days/week:** Campus gym strength training - 45 minutes

- **3 days/week:** Cardio (running, elliptical, group fitness classes) - 30-45 minutes

- **1 day/week:** Active recovery (intramural sports, hiking)

Expected Progress:

- **Weeks 1-2:** 2-3 lbs (1-1.4kg) loss

- **Weeks 3-16:** 1-1.5 lbs (0.5-0.7kg) loss per week

- **Final result:** 20 lbs (9kg) lost in 4-5 months

Key Success Strategies:

- Use campus gym during off-peak hours

- Find dining hall options that fit macros

- Join active clubs or intramural sports

ROBERT - The Retirement Reboot *Age: 58 | Current: 200 lbs (97kg) | Goal: 770 lbs (77kg) | Timeline: 70-12 months*

Robert recently retired and wants to get in the best shape of his life. He has time to focus on health but needs to account for age-related muscle loss and a slower metabolism.

Daily Nutrition Plan:

- **Protein Target:** 170-204 grams (6-7.2 oz) per day (higher due to age)

- **Calories:** 1,700-1,800 per day

- **Breakfast:** 4-egg omelet with vegetables and 2 slices turkey bacon (35g protein, 400 calories)

- **Lunch:** Large salad with 6 oz (170g) grilled salmon and avocado (40g protein, 500 calories)

- **Dinner:** 6 oz (170g) lean beef with roasted vegetables and quinoa (45g protein, 550 calories)

- **Snacks:** Greek yogurt with nuts, protein shake (30g protein, 300 calories total)

Daily Exercise (60-75 minutes):

- **4 days/week:** Strength training (focus on major muscle groups) - 45 minutes

- **3 days/week:** Low-impact cardio (walking, swimming, cycling) - 45 minutes

- **Daily:** 10-minute morning walk

Expected Progress:

- **Weeks 1-2:** 2-3 lbs (1-1.4kg) loss

- **Weeks 3-40:** 0.75-1 lb (0.3-0.5kg) loss per week (slower due to age)

- **Final result:** 30 lbs (14kg) lost in 10-11 months, significant muscle gain

Key Success Strategies:

- Focus on resistance training to combat age-related muscle loss

- Regular health check-ups to monitor progress safely

- Join senior fitness groups for accountability

AMANDA - The Young Professional *Age: 28* | *Current: 740 lbs (64kg)* | *Goal: Build muscle, maintain weight* | *Timeline: Ongoing*

Amanda is already at a healthy weight but wants to build lean muscle and improve her body composition. She's willing to eat more and lift weights but doesn't want to gain fat.

Daily Nutrition Plan:

- **Protein Target:** 140-168 grams (4.9-5.9 oz) per day

- **Calories:** 1,900-2,100 per day (higher for muscle building)

- **Breakfast:** Protein pancakes made with protein powder, oats, and egg whites (35g protein, 400 calories)

- **Lunch:** Quinoa bowl with 5 oz (140g) chicken, vegetables, and tahini (40g protein, 550 calories)

- **Dinner:** 5 oz (140g) white fish with sweet potato and green vegetables (35g protein, 500 calories)

- **Snacks:** Post-workout protein shake, Greek yogurt with nuts (30g protein, 400 calories total)

Daily Exercise (60-75 minutes):

- **4 days/week:** Progressive strength training (compound movements focus) - 60 minutes

- **2 days/week:** Light cardio or yoga - 30 minutes

- **1 day/week:** Complete rest

Expected Progress:

- **Weeks 1-4:** Body recomposition begins (scale weight stable)

- **Months 2-6:** 3-5 lbs (1.4-2.3kg) muscle gain, 3-5 lbs (1.4-2.3kg) fat loss

- **Final result:** Stronger, leaner appearance at same or slightly higher weight

Key Success Strategies:

- Track progress with photos and measurements, not just scale

- Progressive overload in strength training

- Adequate rest and recovery

CARLOS - The Weekend Warrior *Age: 35* | *Current: 785 lbs (84kg)* | *Goal: 765 lbs (75kg)* | *Timeline: 5-6 months*

Carlos plays recreational sports on weekends but sits at a desk all week. He wants to lose 20 pounds (9kg) while maintaining his athletic performance.

Daily Nutrition Plan:

- **Protein Target:** 115-132 grams (4 1-4.7 oz) per day

- **Calories:** 1,600-1,700 per day (higher on sports days)

- **Weekday meals:** Focus on lean proteins, vegetables, minimal processed carbs

- **Weekend sports days:** Add 200-300 calories from healthy carbs (oatmeal, fruit, sweet potato)

- **Post-game:** Protein shake within 2 hours of playing

Daily Exercise:
- **3 weekdays:** 30-minute high-intensity circuit training or running

- **1 weekday:** Active recovery (walking, light yoga)

- **Weekends:** Sports (soccer, basketball, tennis) - 90-120 minutes

- **1 weekend day:** Rest

Expected Progress:

- **Weeks 1-2:** 2-3 lbs (1-1.4kg) loss

- **Weeks 3-20:** 1 lb (0.5kg) loss per week

- **Final result:** 20 lbs (9kg) lost in 5-6 months, maintained athletic performance

Key Success Strategies:

- Time carbs around sports activities

- Hydrate extra on game days

- Don't let weekend social eating derail weekly progress

LISA - The Empty Nester *Age: 52* | *Current: 775 lbs (79kg)* | *Goal: 750 lbs (68kg)* | *Timeline: 8-70 months*

Lisa's kids have left home, and she wants to focus on herself. She's dealing with perimenopause symptoms and finds weight loss harder than it used to be.

Daily Nutrition Plan:

- **Protein Target:** 150-180 grams (5.3-6.4 oz) per day (higher for hormone support)

- **Calories:** 1,500-1,600 per day

- **Focus:** Anti-inflammatory foods, adequate healthy fats for hormone production

- **Timing:** Larger breakfast and lunch, lighter dinner

- **Supplements:** Consider vitamin D, omega-3s after consulting doctor

Daily Exercise (50-60 minutes):

- **3 days/week:** Strength training (crucial for bone density) - 45 minutes

- **3 days/week:** Moderate cardio (walking, swimming) - 40 minutes

- **1 day/week:** Yoga or stretching for stress management

Expected Progress:

- **Weeks 1-2:** 1-2 lbs (0.5-0.9kg) loss (slower due to hormones)
- **Weeks 3-36:** 0.75-1 lb (0.3-0.5kg) loss per week

- **Final result:** 25 lbs (11kg) lost in 8-10 months

Key Success Strategies:

- Prioritize sleep and stress management

- Work with healthcare provider on hormone optimization

- Be patient - perimenopause makes everything slower

TYLER - The Teenage Transformation *Age:* 76 |

Current: 780 lbs (82kg) | *Goal: 760 lbs (73kg)* |
Timeline: 6-8 months

Tyler loves video games, pizza, and hanging out with friends. He's been teased about his weight and wants to lose 20 pounds (9kg) but doesn't want to give up all his favorite foods or spend hours in a gym.

Daily Nutrition Plan:

- **Protein Target:** 112-128 grams (4-4.5 oz) per day

- **Calories:** 2,000-2,200 per day (higher due to teenage metabolism and growth)

- **Breakfast:** Protein smoothie with chocolate protein powder, banana, peanut butter, milk (35g protein, 450 calories) - tastes like a milkshake!

- **Lunch:** Homemade "healthier" pizza on whole wheat tortilla with lots of cheese and pepperoni (25g protein, 500 calories)

- **Dinner:** Taco night with lean ground

turkey, cheese, beans, and fun toppings
(30g protein, 550 calories)

- **Snacks:** Greek yogurt with granola, string
cheese with crackers, chocolate milk (22g
protein, 400 calories total)

Fun Foods Strategy:

- **Pizza Fridays:** Make personal pizzas at home with family - still pizza, but with better ingredients

- **Movie snacks:** Air-popped popcorn with parmesan cheese instead of candy

- **Fast food hacks:** Chipotle bowls, Subway with extra meat, In-N-Out protein style burgers

- **Gaming fuel:** Trail mix with dark chocolate, protein bars that taste like candy bars

Daily Exercise (45-60 minutes) - Family Fun Focus:

- **3 days/week:** Family activities - basketball in driveway, hiking, bike rides, rock climbing gym (45-60 minutes)

- **2 days/week:** Active video games - Just Dance, Ring Fit Adventure, VR games (30 minutes)

- **2 days/week:** Sports with friends - pickup basketball, soccer, skateboarding, swimming

Parent Partnership Activities:

- **Cooking together:** Learn to make healthier versions of favorite foods

- **Active competitions:** Family step challenges, weekend adventure outings

- **Grocery shopping:** Learn to read labels and find "better" versions of favorite snacks

- **Meal prep parties:** Make a week's worth of grab-and-go snacks together

Expected Progress:

- **Weeks 1-2:** 2-3 lbs (1-1.4kg) loss

- **Weeks 3-24:** 0.75-1 lb (0.3-0.Skg) loss per week (accounting for continued growth)

- **Final result:** 20 lbs (9kg) lost in 6-8 months, plus increased height and muscle

Key Success Strategies:

- **No forbidden foods:** Just better versions and appropriate portions

- **Make it social:** Include friends and family in healthy activities

- **Focus on addition, not subtraction:** Add protein and vegetables rather than restricting everything

- **Celebrate non-scale victories:** Better energy for sports, clothes fitting better, feeling stronger

Special Considerations for Teens:

- **Still growing:** Don't restrict calories too severely

- **Social life matters:** Plan for pizza parties, movie nights, and friend hangouts

- **School schedule:** Pack portable protein snacks for after school and sports

- **Independence building:** Learn life skills like cooking and grocery shopping

Tyler's plan proves that getting healthier doesn't mean giving up fun or becoming a social outcast. It's about making better choices most of the time while still enjoying being a teenager.

Your Personal Plan

Use these profiles as starting points, but remember that everyone's body responds differently. The key principles remain the same:

1. **Adequate protein based on target weight**

2. **Consistent calorie deficit for fat loss**

3. **Regular resistance training to preserve/build muscle**

4. **Realistic timelines - 1-2 lbs (0.5-0.9kg) per week maximum**

5. **Flexibility to accommodate your real life**

Adjust the specific foods, exercise types, and timelines based on your preferences, schedule, and how your body responds. The goal is sustainable progress, not perfection.

Chapter 16: Making It Stick - The Psychology of Lasting Change

This chapter addresses the mental and emotional aspects of successful body transformation, providing strategies for building sustainable habits and overcoming the psychological barriers that derail most diet attempts.

Changing your body composition isn't just about knowing what to eat and how to exercise. If it were that simple, everyone would be in great shape. The real challenge is the mental game - building new habits, staying motivated through plateaus, and creating sustainable changes that last years, not months.

Why Most Diets Fail: The Psychology

According to research from UCLA, 95% of diets fail within 2-5 years. This isn't because people lack willpower or because the methods don't work. It's because most approaches ignore the psychological and behavioral aspects of change.

The common failure patterns:

All-or-Nothing Thinking: You're either "on" the

diet perfectly or you've "blown it" completely. One cookie becomes a whole sleeve, one missed workout becomes a week off.

Restriction Rebellion: The more you tell yourself you "can't" have something, the more you want it. Eventually, willpower breaks down and you overindulge.

External Motivation Dependence: Relying on scale numbers, compliments from others, or fitting into specific clothes. When these external rewards don't come quickly enough, motivation crashes.

Perfectionist Paralysis: Waiting for the "perfect" time to start, or giving up when life inevitably interferes with perfect execution.

Identity Mismatch: Trying to maintain behaviors that don't match your self-image. If you see yourself as "not an exercise person," you'll unconsciously sabotage exercise habits.

Building Anti-Fragile Habits

Instead of rigid rules that break under pressure, build flexible habits that get stronger when challenged:

The 80/20 Approach: Aim to make optimal choices

80% of the time. The other 20% allows for real life - birthday parties, work dinners, vacation, or just days when you need pizza. This builds sustainability into your plan from the beginning.

Minimum Effective Habits: Identify the smallest version of each habit that still provides benefit:

- Can't do a 30-minute workout? Do 10 minutes
- Can't meal prep for the week? Prep just tomorrow's lunch
- Can't avoid all processed food? Choose the one with the best ingredients

Stack New Habits onto Existing Ones: Use habits you already do consistently as anchors for new behaviors:

- "After I pour my morning coffee, I will eat 30g of protein"
- "After I brush my teeth at night, I will do 2 minutes of stretching"
- "After I sit down at my desk, I will drink a full glass of water"

The Identity-Based Change Model

Instead of focusing on outcomes (lose 20 pounds), focus on identity (become someone who takes care of their health):

Outcome-focused: "I want to lose weight"

Identity-focused: "I want to become someone who prioritizes their health"

Outcome-focused: "I need to exercise more"

Identity-focused: "I am someone who moves their body daily"

Outcome-focused: "I should eat better" **Identity-focused:** "I am someone who nourishes their body with quality food"

Every action you take is a vote for the type of person you want to become. Each healthy meal, each workout, each good choice reinforces your new identity.

Managing the Motivation Rollercoaster

Motivation is unreliable. It comes and goes based on mood, stress, sleep, and countless other factors. Successful people don't rely on motivation - they rely on systems.

The Habit Loop:

1. **Cue:** Environmental trigger that starts the behavior

2. **Routine:** The behavior itself

3. **Reward:** The benefit you get from the behavior

Example Habit Loop for Morning Exercise:

- **Cue:** Alarm goes off at 6 AM

- **Routine:** 20-minute bodyweight workout

- **Reward:** Energy boost and sense of accomplishment

Make the Cue Obvious:

- Lay out workout clothes the night before

- Put protein powder next to coffee maker

- Set phone reminders for meal times

Make the Routine Easy:

- Start with 10-minute workouts, not 60-minute ones

- Prep grab-and-go protein snacks

- Choose exercises you can do at home

Make the Reward Satisfying:

- Track workouts completed, not just weight lost

- Celebrate consistency milestones

- Focus on how you feel, not just how you look

Dealing with Setbacks and Plateaus

Setbacks aren't failures - they're learning opportunities. Everyone who successfully transforms their body experiences multiple setbacks along the way.

The Bounce-Back Protocol:

1. **Acknowledge without judgment:** "I overate this weekend" not "I'm a failure"

2. **Identify the trigger:** Was it stress? Social pressure? Lack of planning?

3. **Adjust the system:** How can you handle this situation better next time?

4. **Get back on track immediately:** The next meal, not next Monday

Breaking Through Plateaus: Weight loss plateaus are normal and expected. Your body adapts to your new habits and becomes more efficient.

Plateau strategies:

- Take progress photos and measurements, not just scale weight

- Reassess calorie needs as your weight drops

- Add variety to exercise routine

- Take a planned diet break at maintenance calories for 1-2 weeks

- Focus on non-scale victories (energy, sleep, strength, mood)

The Social Environment Factor

Your environment has enormous influence on your success. Research shows that you're more likely to be overweight if your close friends are overweight, and more likely to be fit if your close friends are fit.

Optimize Your Environment:

- Stock your kitchen with healthy options

- Remove or hide tempting processed foods

- Find workout partners or accountability buddies

- Join communities (online or offline) with similar health goals

- Communicate your goals to supportive family and friends

Handle Social Pressure:

- Have responses ready for people pushing food: "Thanks, I'm good for now"

- Suggest active social activities instead of food-centered ones

- Don't make your healthy choices a topic of conversation

- Lead by example, don't preach to others

The Long-Term Mindset

Successful body transformation requires thinking in years, not weeks. This mindset shift changes everything:

Short-term thinking: "I need to lose 20 pounds by summer" **Long-term thinking:** "I want to build habits that keep me healthy for decades"

Short-term thinking: "This plateau means my plan isn't working" **Long-term thinking:** "Plateaus are normal parts of the process"

Short-term thinking: "I messed up this weekend, so I'll start over Monday" **Long-term thinking:** "One weekend doesn't define my overall progress"

Maintenance Planning

Most people focus all their energy on losing weight and zero energy on maintaining the loss. This is backwards. Maintenance is where you'll spend most of your time.

Start practicing maintenance behaviors now:

- Develop sustainable exercise routines you can do long-term
- Learn to navigate social situations without

derailing progress

- Build flexibility into your eating patterns

- Develop non-food stress management strategies

- Create identity and habits, not just rules and restrictions

The Self-Compassion Advantage

Research consistently shows that people who treat themselves with compassion during setbacks are more likely to achieve long-term success than those who use harsh self-criticism.

Self-compassion in practice:

- Talk to yourself like you would talk to a good friend

- Recognize that setbacks and struggles are normal human experiences

- Focus on learning and improvement, not perfection

- Celebrate small wins and progress, not just final outcomes

Your Personal Success System

Create your own success system using these elements:

Daily Habits (non-negotiable minimums):

- One protein-rich meal

- 10 minutes of movement

- One vegetable serving

Weekly Practices:

- Meal planning or prep session

- Progress assessment (photos, measurements, or fitness test)

- Social connection with supportive people

Monthly Reviews:

- What's working well?

- What needs adjustment?

- How is your identity evolving?

- What obstacles can you anticipate and plan for?

The Bottom Line on Psychology

Your body transformation will succeed or fail based on the habits you build and the mindset you maintain. Focus more energy on the psychological aspects of change and less on finding the "perfect" diet or workout plan.

Remember: you're not just trying to lose weight or build muscle. You're becoming the type of person who takes care of their health. That identity shift, supported by sustainable habits and a long-term mindset, is what separates temporary changes from permanent transformation.

Chapter 17: Your Journey Starts Now - Why You'll Succeed When Others Don't

This final chapter recaps the key principles from the book while providing an inspiring framework for long-term success, community building, and understanding why persistence beats perfection in lasting body transformation.

You now have something most people never get: a complete, science-based roadmap for transforming your body without gimmicks, extremes, or unsustainable restrictions. But knowledge alone isn't enough. The difference between success and failure lies in application, persistence, and the courage to keep going when progress feels slow.

The Simple Truth About Success

After 16 chapters of detailed science and practical strategies, the fundamentals of success come down to four principles:

1. **Eat adequate protein based on your target weight** (0.7-1.2g per pound/1.6-2.6g per kg)

2. **Create a moderate calorie deficit through food choices and daily movement**

3. **Do resistance training 3-4 times per week, even if it's just bodyweight exercises at home**

4. **Be patient and consistent for months, not weeks**

That's it. Everything else in this book is optimization and troubleshooting around these four core principles.

Why Most Programs Fail (And Why Yours Won't)

The $70 billion weight loss industry has a dirty secret: they profit from your failure. Quick fixes, dramatic promises, and before-and-after photos sell products, but they don't create lasting change.

Here's why typical programs fail:

They promise too much too fast. "Lose 30 pounds in 30 days!" sounds appealing, but rapid weight loss is mostly water and muscle, not fat. You end up with a slower metabolism and regain the weight quickly.

They're too restrictive. Eliminating entire food groups or requiring perfect adherence to complicated rules works for a few weeks, then real life intervenes. One "mistake" turns into complete abandonment.

They ignore the psychology. Focusing only on what to eat and how to exercise while ignoring habits, mindset, and social factors sets people up for failure.

They have an endpoint. "Do this for 12 weeks" implies you can go back to old habits afterward. Sustainable results require sustainable changes.

They're one-size-fits-all. A plan designed for a 25-year-old male athlete won't work for a 45-year-old working mother, but most programs ignore individual circumstances.

Why Your Approach Will Succeed

You're playing the long game. You understand that meaningful change takes 6-12 months, not 6-12 weeks. This mindset alone puts you ahead of 90% of people who start transformation journeys.

You have flexible, evidence-based guidelines, not rigid rules. You can adapt these principles to any lifestyle, culture, or preference while maintaining effectiveness.

You're building identity and habits, not following a temporary diet. You're becoming someone who prioritizes their health, not someone who's temporarily restricting food.

You understand that imperfection is part of the process. Progress beats perfection. Consistency beats intensity. Small improvements compounded over time beat dramatic short-term changes.

You have realistic expectations. Losing 1-2 pounds (0.5-0.9kg) per week isn't glamorous, but it's sustainable and maintainable.

The Power of Persistence

Every person who has successfully transformed their body and maintained it long-term has one trait in common: they didn't quit when things got difficult.

You will face challenges:

- Weeks when the scale doesn't move despite perfect adherence

- Social situations that test your resolve

- Injuries or illnesses that disrupt your routine

- Life stress that makes healthy choices harder

- Moments when you question whether it's worth the effort

This is normal. These challenges don't mean you're failing or that the approach doesn't work. They mean you're human, living a real life, dealing with real obstacles.

The people who succeed are not the ones who never face challenges. They're the ones who keep going despite challenges.

Your Success Network: Finding Your Tribe

One of the strongest predictors of long-term success is having social support from people with similar goals. You need people who understand what you're trying to accomplish and can provide encouragement when motivation wanes.

Where to find your support network:

Online Communities:

- Reddit communities like r/loseit, r/fitness, r/bodyweightfitness

- Facebook groups focused on sustainable weight loss

- Apps like MyFitnessPal that have social features

- Instagram hashtags like #sustainableweightloss #strengthtraining

Local Options:

- Walking groups or hiking clubs

- Community center fitness classes

- Recreational sports leagues

- Cooking classes focused on healthy eating

- Local CrossFit boxes or yoga studios

Family and Friends: Don't underestmate the power of recruiting existing relationships. Share your goals with supportive people in your life and ask for specific help:

- "Can we try cooking healthy meals together?"

- "Would you be my walking partner a few times per week?"

- "Can you help me stay accountable by checking in monthly?"

Workplace Wellness: Many employers have wellness programs or groups. Starting a workplace walking club or healthy potluck group can provide both social support and convenient timing.

What to Look For in Support Partners:

Similar goals but different strengths. You don't need people exactly like you. Someone further along can provide inspiration and advice. Someone just starting can provide mutual encouragement.

Positive, non-judgmental attitudes. Avoid groups that shame "bad" foods or promote extreme behaviors. Look for communities that celebrate progress and acknowledge setbacks as normal.

Focus on health, not just appearance. While looking better is a valid goal, groups that also emphasize strength, energy, and overall health tend to be more sustainable and supportive.

Realistic timelines and expectations. Avoid groups promoting quick fixes or comparing themselves to social media transformations.

The Marathon Mindset

Think of your body transformation like training for a marathon, not sprinting a 100-meter dash.

Month 1-2: Building the Foundation You're learning new habits, establishing routines, and seeing initial changes. Motivation is high, results are encouraging. Enjoy this phase but don't expect it to last forever.

Month 3-6: The Middle Miles Progress slows down. Habits are forming but not automatic yet. This is where most people quit. Push through. This phase is building the psychological strength that will sustain you long-term.

Month 6-12: Finding Your Rhythm Healthy choices

become more automatic. You've navigated challenges and built confidence. Progress is steady but not dramatic. You're becoming the person you wanted to be.

Year 2 and Beyond: Lifestyle Integration Your healthy habits are now part of who you are. You've learned to navigate holidays, vacations, stress, and life changes while maintaining your progress. You're no longer "on a diet" - you're living a healthy lifestyle.

Your Personal Mission Statement

Before you close this book, take a moment to write your personal mission statement. This isn't about weight loss goals or appearance targets. It's about the deeper reasons you want to change and the person you want to become

Fill in these blanks:

"I am committed to taking care of my health because…

"Six months from now …

"When I face challenges, I will remember that ...

"My definition of success includes ...

Examples:

- "I am committed to taking care of my health because I want to have energy to play with my grandchildren."

- "Six months from now, I will be someone who prioritizes movement and nourishing food without guilt or obsession."

- "When I face challenges, I will remember that every healthy choice is a vote for the person I'm becoming."

- "My definition of success includes feeling strong, sleeping well, and having a healthy relationship with food."

The Ripple Effect

Your transformation won't just affect you. When you become healthier, stronger, and more confident, it impacts everyone around you:

- Your children learn that taking care of your body is normal and important

- Your friends see that sustainable change is possible

- Your coworkers notice your increased energy and positivity

- Your family benefits from healthier meals and

more active lifestyle choices

You're not just changing your body - you're becoming an example of what's possible when someone commits to their health with patience and consistency.

Your Next Steps

1. **Choose your starting point.** Review the profiles in Chapter 15 and pick the one most similar to your situation. Use it as a template, but adjust based on your preferences and schedule.

2. **Set up your environment.** Stock your kitchen with protein sources and vegetables. Clear space for home workouts. Download a food tracking app if helpful.

3. **Find your people.** Identify at least one source of social support, whether online or in person.

4. **Start small but start today.** Don't wait for Monday, or next month, or when you have everything figured out. Do one thing today that moves you toward your goal.

5. **Commit to the process, not just the outcome.** Focus on building habits and identity, trusting that the physical changes will follow.

The Truth About Transformation

Real transformation isn't about willpower, perfection, or dramatic overhauls. It's about making slightly better choices, consistently, over time. It's about progress, not perfection. It's about becoming someone who takes care of their health because that's who they are, not because they're following a temporary plan.

You have everything you need to succeed. The science is clear, the methods are proven, and the path is laid out in front of you. The only question is whether you'll take the first step, and then the second, and then the third.

Your journey starts now. Not when you finish reading this book, not when you have more time, not when life gets easier. Now.

You've got this. Your future self is counting on the choices you make today. Make them count.

Welcome to the beginning of the rest of your life.

Printed in France by Amazon
Brétigny-sur-Orge, FR

40225488R00090